Fluid
Vete
Techn...uians

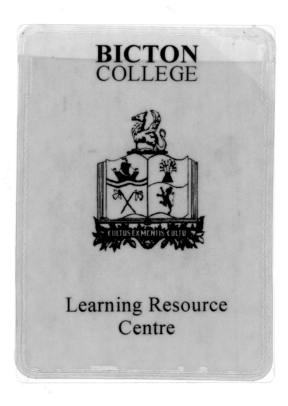

BICTON
COLLEGE

CULTUS EX MENTIS CULTU

Learning Resource
Centre

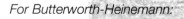

For Butterworth-Heinemann:

Commissioning Editor: *Mary Seager*
Development Editor: *Catharine Steers*
Project Managers: *Pat Miller; Gail Wright*
Designer: *Andy Chapman*

Fluid Therapy for Veterinary Nurses and Technicians

Paula Hotston Moore VN
Vetlink School of Veterinary Nursing Ltd, Yeovil, UK

Foreword by

Andrea Jeffery CertEd DipAVN(Surg) VN
Tutor in Veterinary Nursing, Department of Clinical Veterinary Science,
University of Bristol, Bristol, UK

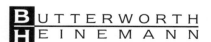

BUTTERWORTH
HEINEMANN

EDINBURGH LONDON NEW YORK OXFORD PHILADELPHIA ST LOUIS SYDNEY TORONTO 2004

BUTTERWORTH-HEINEMANN
An imprint of Elsevier Science Limited

First published 2004

ISBN 0 7506 5283 7

British Library Cataloguing in Publication Data
A catalogue record for this book is available from the British Library

Library of Congress Cataloging in Publication Data
A catalog record for this book is available from the Library of Congress

Notice
Veterinary knowledge is constantly changing. Standard safety precautions
must be followed, but as new research and clinical experience broaden our
knowledge, changes in treatment and drug therapy may become necessary
or appropriate. Readers are advised to check the most current product
information provided by the manufacturer of each drug to be administered to
verify the recommended dose, the method and duration of administration,
and contraindications. It is the responsibility of the practitioner, relying on
experience and knowledge of the patient, to determine dosages and the best
treatment for each individual patient. Neither the Publisher nor the Author
assumes any liability for any injury and/or damage to persons or property
arising from this publication.

The Publisher

your source for books,
journals and multimedia
in the health sciences
www.elsevierhealth.com

The
Publisher's
policy is to use
**paper manufactured
from sustainable forests**

Printed in China

Contents

Foreword

Fluid therapy is one area of patient treatment in which veterinary nurses need to have the fullest confidence and knowledge to enable them to carry out the procedures and nursing care involved correctly, and indeed the RCVS Veterinary Nursing Syllabus and Occupational Standards reflect nurses' need for this knowledge.

This book is therefore timely in offering a comprehensive insight into fluid therapy and the nurse's role in carrying this out effectively and responsibly. It will be of value to students and qualified nurses alike since the layout allows it to be used as a revision aid as well as a quick reference guide. I am happy to recommend it as a book that should be kept on the shelf in the hospitalisation areas of all veterinary practices.

Andrea Jeffery

Preface

Fluid therapy is vital in the treatment and support of many conditions in animals. It involves practical nursing care as well as a good theoretical knowledge of *why* an animal needs fluid administration, the *choice* of fluid to be given and *how* that fluid is to be administered. In this book, my aim has been to outline these key areas by offering some insight to the theory involved, and by considering the practicalities of fluid administration and patient monitoring.

Veterinary nurses administer fluid therapy under the supervision of a veterinary surgeon, but they will obtain greater professional satisfaction if they also have the underpinning knowledge as to why a particular fluid is given, as well as prior knowledge of any potential problems that could arise.

This book provides a comprehensive and structured account of many aspects of fluid therapy but is also designed to allow veterinary nurses to 'dip in' to specific areas as needed to refresh their knowledge or answer a particular clinical problem. Until now, there has not been a book aimed at veterinary nurses that is dedicated to the subject of fluid therapy alone. My aim has been to fill that gap!

Shipham 2003   Paula Hotston Moore

Acknowledgements

I would like to thank Alasdair for his help and support in the writing of this book. I would like to thank all student veterinary nurses, past and present, who have helped me realise the need for a book on fluid therapy. I hope this helps them both in their training and after! Finally, I would like to thank Esme and Alice for putting up with sharing my time between this book and them!

1

Water and electrolyte balance in the body

Key points

- Water comprises 60–70% of bodyweight
- Fluid in the body exists in several different 'compartments', and can move between these to help correct losses or imbalances
- Electrolytes within body fluid are important for normal cell and organ function
- Shock results when the circulatory system cannot deliver adequate oxygen to tissues and organs; this often happens as a result of body fluid disturbances, e.g. loss of fluid through bleeding
- Fluid therapy, and subsequent monitoring, is vital in the treatment of shock

Body water

Water is vital for normal cellular function in the body. Between 60–70% of a healthy animal's bodyweight comprises water, which is made available to the animal in three ways: through diet, drinking water and as a consequence of metabolic processes which release water from certain nutrients.

The major source of body water is through drinking. The amount an animal drinks depends upon the availability of the drinking water and the type of diet the animal is fed on. Behaviour also plays a role: some animals prefer to drink from streams, pots of water in the garden or other sources. When these are available, the owner may not notice much water being taken from indoor drinking bowls, resulting in a low apparent water intake. If these sources of water were prevented or removed, visible water intake would increase. Such behavioural habits or preferences must be borne in mind when trying to assess water intake.

Water also enters the animal's body through the diet, and this depends on the composition of the food being fed, i.e. dry or wet (tinned/fresh). The metabolism of fat and carbohydrates also produces some water in the animal's body.

The body loses water in three main ways: urinary loss, faecal loss and 'inevitable' loss. Inevitable losses are those that the animal has no control over: respiratory and cutaneous losses. Water is lost from the respiratory tract during normal respiration because, during inhalation and exhalation, evaporation of fluid occurs in the lining of the respiratory passages and in the mouth. Cutaneous losses help cool the body through evaporation of water via sweat glands (also known as sudoriferous glands).

The figures in Box 1.1 are a rough estimate of how much fluid is lost from an animal over a 24 hour period. The usual estimate of fluid loss is 50–60 mL/kg/24 hours based on these figures. In the normal healthy animal, water intake and water output are equal. Note that puppies and

---

Box 1.1   Normal water losses from the body

Faecal losses:	10–20 mL/kg/24 hours
Urinary losses:	20 mL/kg/24 hours
Inevitable losses:	20 mL/kg/24 hours
Total losses:	50–60 mL/kg/24 hours

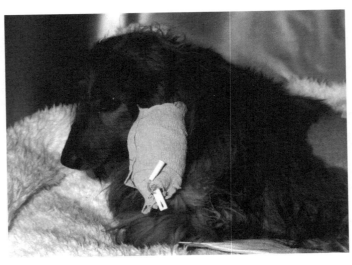

Figure 1.1 Intravenous catheterisation of the ear vein. Secure bandaging is necessary to keep this catheter in place.

kittens have a higher maintenance fluid requirement than adults: up to 80 mL/kg/24 hours. This is partly due to their reduced ability to concentrate urine, hence higher urinary loss is incurred.

Since the normal adult healthy animal loses 50–60 mL/kg/24 hours, the same amount of fluid needs to be taken into the body in order to maintain a balance. We say then that the animal needs 50–60 mL/kg/24 hours to balance its intake and losses of water over a 24 hour period. This is known as the **maintenance requirement.**

Body fluid compartments

Approximately 60% of bodyweight is fluid. Realistically, this means that just over half the weight of a dog or cat is made up of fluid! When we think about it in this way, we begin to realise why fluid therapy is so important. In young and lean animals slightly more of their bodyweight is fluid: approximately 70%. In geriatric and obese animals, slightly less is fluid: approximately 50% of body weight.

The fluid in the body is distributed in certain specific areas. 40% of fluid is inside the cells of the body – this is called *intracellular fluid* (ICF) and represents the largest fluid compartment in the body. The remaining 20% of fluid is outside the cells of the body – this is called *extracellular fluid* (ECF).

Extracellular fluid is found in three places:

- Plasma water
- Interstitial fluid
- Transcellular fluid.

Fluid inside the blood vessels is termed *plasma water* (PW) or *intravascular fluid* and makes up 5% of the extracellular fluid; plasma water suspends the blood cells in blood vessels. There is fluid around the tissue cells of the body, which is termed *interstitial fluid* (ISF); this makes up 15% of the extracellular fluid. A small amount of fluid is found in places such as the subdural space (cerebrospinal fluid) and the synovial cavities (synovial fluid). This is termed *transcellular fluid* (TCF); less than 1% of extracellular fluid is found as transcellular fluid.

Figure 1.2 shows the distribution of water in the body.

Semipermeable membranes and electrolytes

The major fluid compartments are separated by a semipermeable membrane, which allows fluid to pass freely between each compartment. Water will pass through a semipermeable membrane to follow certain dissolved substances, especially the electrolytes sodium, potassium and

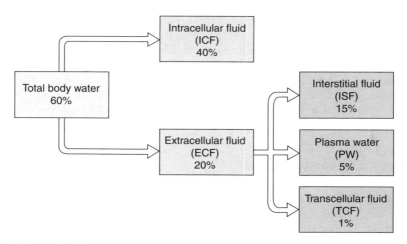

Figure 1.2 Body fluids as a percentage of bodyweight, and their distribution in the various compartments.

Table 1.1	The composition of body fluids		
	Plasma water (mmol/L)	Interstitial fluid (mmol/L)	Intracellular fluid (mmol/L)
Cations			
Sodium (Na^+)	142	145	10
Potassium (K^+)	4	4	150
Calcium (Ca^{++})	2.5	2.4	4
Magnesium (Mg^{++})	1	1	34
Anions			
Chloride (Cl^-)	104	117	4
Bicarbonate (HCO_3^-)	24	27	12

magnesium. In each fluid compartment in the body the amount of these substances differs, hence the amount of water in these compartments also differs. The principal electrolytes in extracellular fluid are sodium, chloride and bicarbonate. Electrolytes in intracellular fluid consist mainly of potassium and magnesium (Table 1.1).

Cell membranes are permeable to sodium. A pump, the ATPase pump, is situated on the cell membrane and removes any sodium that tends to leak into the cell, exchanging it for potassium. Adenosine triphosphate (ATP) is used as the energy source to pump sodium out of the cell, hence the pump's name. There is more potassium inside

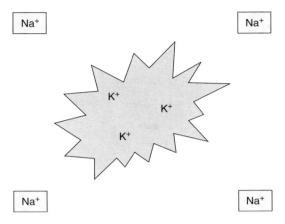

Figure 1.3 Potassium is maintained inside the cell, and sodium outside, by the action of the sodium or ATPase pump.

the cell than on the outside and the action of the pump maintains this balance (Fig. 1.3).

As explained earlier (and shown in Fig. 1.2), the fluid compartments in the body are not all the same size. This means that fluid loss from a small body compartment (such as the plasma water or blood vessels) will have a much greater effect than similar fluid loss taken from a larger body compartment (such as the intracellular fluid). The larger intracellular compartment is able to accommodate the loss much more easily. As a simple analogy, compare this to having a thimbleful or a pint of beer. A sip taken from the thimbleful will probably nearly empty it, but one taken from the pint will be barely noticeable. The loss from the thimbleful is therefore much more significant.

In reality, when fluid is lost from an animal, the body always strives to ensure that the loss is evenly distributed throughout the various body fluid compartments. So if fluid is lost from one compartment, water moves across the semipermeable membrane to disperse between the compartments, spreading out the loss or deficit. This ensures that no one compartment is low on fluid whilst the other compartments are all normal.

This also means that when water is lost from the body, some water is lost from *all* compartments as the body attempts to redistribute the remaining fluid. Depending upon the size of the fluid compartment concerned, this may be of greater or lesser importance. Since the plasma water is a small compartment in the first place, any loss here is significant (remember the thimble of beer story!). Figure 1.4 shows fluid movements between compartments of different sizes in the body.

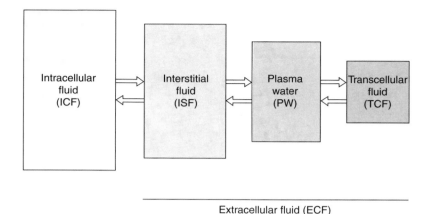

Extracellular fluid (ECF)

Figure 1.4 Fluid movements can occur between compartments of different sizes. Fluid loss from a smaller compartment is always more significant, but can be compensated by influx of fluid from a larger one.

Regulation of changes in body water

Fluid loss from the plasma water compartment has two distinct effects. Firstly, osmoreceptors stimulate the release of antidiuretic hormone and the animal becomes thirsty. Antidiuretic hormone (ADH) promotes the reabsorption of water from the renal tubules and this *increases* the concentration of urine that is passed (thus *decreasing* its volume). Secondly, the kidneys detect a reduction in the plasma water compartment as a reduction in renal blood flow. This stimulates the release of renin, which in turn generates angiotensin. Angiotensin stimulates the release of aldosterone and aldosterone acts on the kidney to increase the reabsorption of sodium within the distal convoluted tubule. Water is reabsorbed too (it follows sodium), resulting in more concentrated urine being passed.

This sequence will also work the other way. If the osmotic concentration of plasma water is reduced (becomes dilute), less antidiuretic hormone is released, less water is reabsorbed in the kidney and the urine becomes more dilute.

Shock

Shock can be defined as acute circulatory collapse. The circulatory system is not able to carry sufficient oxygen and nutrients around the body. If left untreated, reversible shock may progress to severe (irreversible) shock and eventually death.

Signs of shock

The signs of shock are seen in all the organ systems. They include:

- Decreased mental alertness
- Cold, pale, clammy or dry mucous membranes
- Prolonged capillary refill time
- Cyanosis or injected (brick-red) mucous membranes
- Raised heart rate
- Weak, rapid pulse
- Reduced urine output
- Reduced or raised body temperature
- Reduced respiratory rate.

Possible causes of shock

Shock may be caused by the following problems/conditions:

- Haemorrhage, both internal and external
- Prolonged vomiting
- Prolonged diarrhoea
- Central nervous system trauma
- Reaction to a substance (anaphylactic shock)
- Release of endotoxins into the blood stream
- Severe dehydration.

Treatment of shock

The aim of treating shock is to ensure the return of peripheral perfusion (blood flow) to a level adequate for the animal's needs. The cornerstone of this treatment is fluid therapy because, in almost all cases, cardiac output is directly dependent on blood volume. By increasing blood volume we can increase cardiac output and thus increase oxygen delivery and peripheral circulation. Other methods of treatment must be considered secondary to fluid therapy.

Fluid administration

Intravenous fluid therapy is essential. The choice of fluids is important but it has been said that *how much* you give is more important than *what* you give, i.e. in a crisis any fluid is better than no fluid at all.

Initially in severe shock (e.g. when the pulse is barely palpable and the patient is collapsed) Hartmann's (lactated Ringer's) solution is given at a dose of 60 mL/kg as rapidly as possible. This dose rate is equivalent to about 2.5 L for a Labrador or around 250 mL for a cat and requires the placement of a large gauge intravenous catheter, preferably in the jugular vein. If an intravenous catheter cannot be placed due to circulatory collapse, a needle may be used to give fluids into a bone marrow cavity (the intraosseous route).

At this time the packed cell volume (PCV) and plasma protein level should be assessed. If the PCV is less than 25%, whole blood should be given to raise it to this level. If the PCV is higher than 25%, blood is not usually required. If the plasma protein is less than 40 g/L, whole blood or a colloid solution should be given. If this treatment does not restore an adequate pulse or other sign of improvement, it should be repeated and PCV reassessed.

Further investigations and history taking should now commence. If there is evidence or history of heart disease, fluid therapy should now be more cautious – a further 5–10 mL/kg of colloid may be given; in other cases give another 30 mL/kg of Hartmann's. These steps should result in improved pulse and pink mucous membranes. If not, reassess the patient and repeat treatment if required. Assess and treat any other problems such as continued blood loss.

Monitoring

Ideally, during treatment of shock, central venous blood pressure (CVP) should be measured and maintained below 12 cmH₂O. An accumulation of breakdown products can result in excess acidity of the blood (acidosis). This should be automatically corrected with the administration of Hartmann's solution but it can be more rapidly achieved using intravenous sodium bicarbonate solution if severe. Similarly, alterations in blood potassium are common and may need to be corrected.

Adequate urine output should be ensured. Ideally, this is measured and maintained at 1–2 mL/kg/hr by the administration of fluids and other supportive drug therapy.

The body temperature is readily assessed. This should be maintained between 38–39°C by gentle warming or cooling of the patient as required.

Antibiotics should be given when infection is known or suspected, or when shock is severe or prolonged.

Glucose may be needed to be given to maintain a normal blood level. The role of corticosteroids in shock treatment remains controversial. These are often used on the basis that they 'do no harm' – this may or may not be true. If they are to be used rationally, they must be given early and in very high doses, e.g. 5 mg/kg of dexamethasone (e.g. Dexadreson;

Intervet) given intravenously. This dose rate works out at 75 mL for an average Labrador – much more than the doses usually given.

Box 1.2 Summarises basic treatment for a patient with shock.

Box 1.2   Suggested fluid therapy for patients with shock

Step 1   If pulse not palpable, begin cardiopulmonary resuscitation (CPR).

Step 2   If pulse weak or barely palpable, begin intravenous Hartmann's at 60 mL/kg given as rapidly as possible. Check PCV and plasma protein (PP).

Step 3   Monitor central venous pressure (CVP). Stop fluids if exceeds 15 cmH$_2$O.

Step 4   If PCV is less than 25% or plasma protein is less than 40 g/L give blood or plasma expander.

Step 5   Pulse should now be adequate. If not repeat steps 1–4.

Step 6   Obtain further history and begin work-up. Repeat PCV and plasma protein measurement and treat if indicated. Give a further 30 mL/kg of fluids if no history of heart disease, else 5–10 mL/kg of plasma expander.

Step 7   CVP should now be 5–12 cmH$_2$O, pulse strong, CRT less than 2 seconds and mucous membranes pink. If not, repeat steps 6–7.

Step 8   Finish diagnostics. Check for continuing blood loss. Begin maintenance fluids.

2

Assessment of fluid balance

Key points

- The commonest fluid loss in animals is a mixed loss of water and electrolytes

- Assessment and treatment of disturbances in blood electrolyte levels (especially potassium) is an important part of fluid therapy

- Dehydration can be assessed in various ways, including clinical history, clinical examination/measurement and using the results of laboratory tests

- Central venous pressure measurement can be an aid to fluid therapy and monitoring, however the technique is invasive and not commonly performed in practice

Fluid loss

An animal is dehydrated when it has suffered an excessive loss of fluid from the body. Three types of fluid loss or deficit are recognised: primary water loss, mixed electrolyte and water loss, and blood loss. The choice of replacement fluid depends on which type of loss the animal has suffered.

Primary water loss or deficit

A deficit of water only is often caused by a reduction in the animal's daily intake. This may be due to an inability to take in water in situations such as facial trauma, absence of drinking water and general weakness or lethargy. A common cause of water loss is increased excretion, which can occur in clinical conditions such as diabetes insipidus or renal disease. In these situations, the animal has lost (or failed to take in) water only; electrolyte disturbances have not occurred.

Water and electrolyte loss

This is a loss of both water *and* electrolytes from the animal's body. Electrolytes are chemical substances found in the body such as sodium, potassium, magnesium, etc. They are important for normal tissue and organ function. This type of fluid loss is the most common type affecting animals.

There are many clinical situations when the animal will lose both water and electrolytes, e.g. vomiting, diarrhoea, wounds, burns, pyometra, and ascites. In the case of the vomiting animal stomach contents or bile as well as fluid (water) are lost. Stomach contents and bile contain electrolytes so both water and electrolyte loss has occurred. In the animal suffering from diarrhoea, much fluid may be lost in the watery faeces, which, as well as waste products, also contains electrolytes. Again, a mixed loss of water and electrolytes has occurred.

Blood loss

Blood loss occurs in cases of haemorrhage. External haemorrhage is usually apparent but internal haemorrhage must also be considered as considerable volumes of blood may be lost into body cavities such as the abdomen or chest.

Potassium

Potassium is mainly intracellular (see Ch.1, Fig. 1.3), with only a small amount being extracellular. When electrolytes are considered, changes to potassium levels in the body are particularly serious and cause clinical signs such as bradycardia, cardiac arrhythmias and lethargy. If left untreated, these disturbances can be life threatening. By considering the type of fluid loss, we must decide whether the animal is likely to be suffering from potassium depletion (hypokalaemia) or potassium accumulation (hyperkalaemia).

Potassium balance

Potassium is taken into the body with food and is usually lost through excretion by the kidneys. Any disease or trauma affecting these routes will in turn affect the levels of potassium in the body. When fluid is replaced during fluid therapy we must consider potassium levels. If significant potassium has been lost, then this electrolyte must be added to the intravenous fluids; if potassium has been accumulated, we must ensure no more potassium enters the body during fluid therapy. Some fluids used in fluid therapy contain potassium and some do not so the choice can be important.

Since potassium enters the body in food, any condition affecting eating or a low dietary intake could in turn cause potassium depletion. Conditions such as prolonged inappetence, vomiting, prolonged diuretic therapy or prolonged diarrhoea can all result in potassium depletion through either a low intake or an increased loss. Diuretics cause an

---

Box 2.1   Possible causes of potassium accumulation and depletion

Potassium depletion

- Prolonged inappetence
- Vomiting
- Prolonged diuretic therapy
- Prolonged diarrhoea

Potassium accumulation

- Urethral obstruction
- Bladder rupture
- Acute renal failure

---

increased volume of urination and therefore increased losses of potassium. Since potassium is excreted from the body via the kidneys and the urinary tract, any disease, trauma or obstruction affecting these tissues may result in a build up of potassium in the body if urine cannot be voided, e.g. urethral obstruction, bladder rupture and acute renal failure can all lead to potassium accumulation, with serious medical consequences.

In determining which type of fluid has been lost from the animal (water loss, fluid and electrolyte or blood) we must therefore also determine whether the animal may be suffering from depletion or accumulation of potassium since this can affect the choice of rehydration fluid.

Assessing dehydration

Any method used to assess the hydration status of the animal results in a rough estimate, as no method is completely accurate. In practice, four main methods are employed to determine the extent of dehydration.

1. Clinical history

It is possible to estimate fluid requirements from what is believed (via clinical history) to have been lost. Generally accepted values for vomiting and diarrhoea losses are used in calculation, e.g. for each vomit it is estimated that the animal has lost 4 mL/kg of fluid.

If a 10 kg dog has vomited twice we can estimate:

$$4 \, mL \times 10 \, kg \times 2 \, vomits = 80 \, mL \, lost \, in \, total.$$

Similarly, it is estimated that for each episode of diarrhoea the animal has lost 4 mL/kg. So if a 20 kg dog has three episodes of diarrhoea then we can estimate:

$$4 \, mL \times 20 \, kg \times 3 \, episodes = 240 \, mL \, lost \, in \, total.$$

---

2. Clinical examination

Clinical examination can give a crude guide as to the degree of dehydration – this is largely based on the loss of skin elasticity, also known as skin turgor. The skin over the scruff of the neck or the eyelid is tented and, in the normal healthy animal, will fall back into position within 2–3 seconds. In the dehydrated animal the skin will take longer to return to its original position.

Other clinical signs used to determine hydration levels are capillary refill time (CRT), dryness of mucous membranes, sunken eyes, mental depression, general weakness and any signs of shock. Normal capillary refill time is less than 2 seconds. Normal mucous membranes are moist and pink; in the dehydrated patient they become dry and tacky. Eyes appear bright in the healthy animal but can be sunken and dull in the dehydrated patient. The normal patient appears alert and interested in life but the dehydrated patient may become lethargic, disinterested and depressed. Table 2.1 lists the clinical signs associated with various levels of dehydration.

Note that clinical examination is very subjective: I could examine an animal and decide it is 6% dehydrated but you could estimate it to be 10% dehydrated. This is not hugely important since from the clinical examination we only aim to have a *rough* initial guide as to the level of dehydration of the animal.

Table 2.1 Clinical signs associated with different degrees of dehydration

Dehydration (%)	Clinical signs
<5	Not detectable
5–6	Subtle loss of skin elasticity
6–8	Marked loss of skin elasticity Slightly prolonged capillary refill time Slightly sunken eyes Dry mucous membranes
10–12	Tented skin stands in place Capillary refill time >2 seconds Sunken eyes Dry mucous membranes
12–15	Early shock Collapse Death imminent

Consider a 4 kg cat that appears 10% dehydrated on clinical examination. Fluid requirement is worked out in the following way:

$$\frac{10}{100} \times 4 \text{ kg} = 0.4 \text{ kg}$$

We know that 1 kg ≡ 1 L. The cat which is 0.4 kg dehydrated therefore requires 0.4 L of fluid to reverse that dehydration.

3. Laboratory analyses

The following laboratory tests can be used to estimate the amount and nature of fluid losses:

- Packed cell volume (PCV)
- Haemoglobin
- Total plasma protein
- Urea
- Creatinine

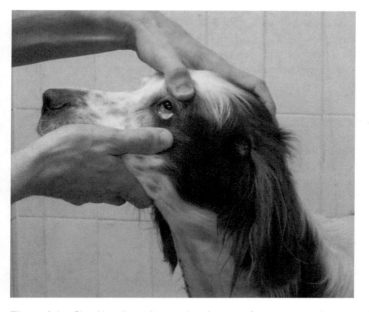

Figure 2.1   Checking the colour and moistness of mucous membranes lining the eyelid to assess hydration. The skin elasticity (turgor) of the eyelid is another useful indicator of degree of dehydration.

- Plasma electrolytes
- Acid–base estimations.

Packed cell volume (PCV) measures the proportion of red blood cells in a centrifuged sample of blood in a capillary tube. It is increased in dehydration since there is a loss of plasma water. Known figures are that for every 1% increase in PCV, a fluid loss of approximately 10 mL/kg has occurred. For this evaluation to be accurate we should know the animal's PCV *prior to* fluid loss. In most cases this information will not be known, therefore a normal PCV of 45% in dogs and 35% in cats is adopted.

> If a 5 kg cat has a PCV of 42% we can calculate as follows: the normal PCV in the cat is 35%; the PCV is now 42%, which is an increase of 7%. So:
>
> $$7\% \times 10\,mL \times 5\,kg = 350\,mL$$
>
> 350 mL fluid is therefore calculated as having been lost.

Haemoglobin levels increase in dehydration since there is a loss of plasma water. Total plasma protein levels also increase in dehydration for the same reason. Packed cell volume taken in conjunction with the total plasma protein level is often used to determine the hydration status of the patient. Plasma urea and creatinine levels are increased in dehydration since there is reduced renal perfusion and hence decreased excretion of these substances.

Electrolytes

Plasma electrolytes can be monitored but this will depend upon the facilities in an individual veterinary practice. To be of value, a blood sample needs to be tested immediately after being taken, so the equipment must be available 'in house'. Often, sodium, potassium and chloride levels are monitored, as the animal that has a fluid imbalance will also likely have an electrolyte imbalance. If possible, base line blood and urine samples should be taken before fluid administration is started so that the response to treatment can be monitored.

4. Clinical measurements

Bodyweight

Measuring **changes in the animal's bodyweight** can give an estimate of how much fluid has been lost in dehydration. For this, the animal's accurate bodyweight *before* dehydration must be known.

We already know that 1 kg ≡ 1 L of fluid. If a 13.5 kg dog weighed 14 kg before it became dehydrated, it has lost 0.5 kg, which equals 0.5 L or 500 mL.

This estimate is not frequently used since many owners are unaware of their pet's weight to a sufficient degree of accuracy. The weight of hospitalised patients is however recorded, so in these cases the calculation can be useful to assess dehydration and response to fluid therapy.

Urine output

Changes in urine output also provide a guide to hydration status. Oliguria (reduced urine output) is present during dehydration. When normal urine output returns this is an indication that fluid replacement is working. Urine output can be monitored by simple observation of the patient or by placement of an indwelling urinary catheter for accurate measurement.

Normal urine output is 1–2 mL/kg/hour.

Central venous pressure

The measurement of **central venous pressure (CVP)** can be used to estimate and monitor hydration status. Central venous pressure is the blood pressure as measured in the right atrium of the heart. The procedure is not often carried out in general veterinary practice since it involves placement of a jugular catheter – a technique that many veterinary surgeons prefer to avoid. There is potential for haemorrhage and severe infection.

The equipment required to monitor central venous pressure is as follows:

- Jugular catheter
- Crystalloid fluid
- Standard fluid giving set
- Three-way tap
- Extension set
- Manometer.

The manometer usually consists of a ruler with a length of extension tubing attached to it along the centimetre scale reading.

The animal is placed in either left lateral or sternal recumbency in order that the right jugular vein is adequately exposed. Either a long 'over-the-needle' or a 'through-the-needle' intravenous catheter is used. The catheter is placed in the jugular vein using strict aseptic technique to prevent contamination. The skin is prepared as if for aseptic surgery, i.e. the hair is widely clipped using a size 40 blade and the skin surface is cleaned with diluted surgical scrub. The surgeon scrubs up and wears sterile gloves for placement of the catheter.

The long catheter is advanced into the right jugular vein until the tip lies almost in the right atrium or vena cava, the catheter having been previously measured from the jugular vein to approximate heart position.

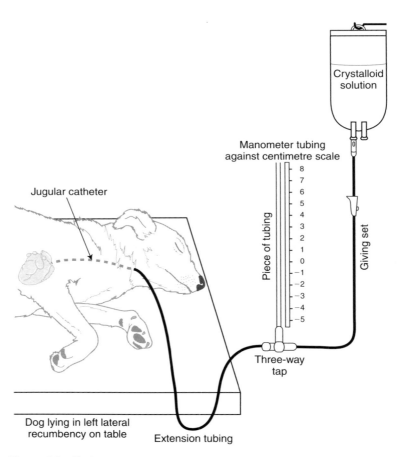

Figure 2.2 Equipment and procedure for measuring central venous pressure in a dog. Pressure is read off the centimetre scale alongside the manometer tubing (see text).

The catheter is then secured (sutured) in place and connected to the central venous pressure monitoring system. The giving set is attached to the bag of crystalloid fluid and a three-way tap connected to the Luer end of the giving set. Also connected to the three-way tap are the extension set and manometer.

Fluid from the bag of crystalloid is run through the giving and extension sets to ensure no air is in the tubing. (This will result in potentially dangerous gas embolism if it reaches the animal.) Fluid is then run through the manometer tubing until level with the zero mark on the centimetre scale. The equipment is now ready to be connected to the jugular catheter. The extension set is connected to the intravenous catheter. The crystalloid fluid is administered to the animal and, by altering the flow direction of fluid via the three-way tap, the central venous pressure can be measured.

To administer fluid to the animal the three-way tap is turned 'off' towards the manometer. To measure central venous pressure the tap is turned 'off' towards the crystalloid fluids. Central venous pressure is measured and recorded on the patient's records. After measurement, fluid is administered to the patient via the giving set, by moving the three-way tap to block the flow to the manometer again. *The animal must be monitored throughout this procedure. The catheter in the jugular vein needs constant supervision: there is potential for life-threatening haemorrhage if it detaches.*

The normal range of central venous pressure is 3–7 cm H_2O. Repeated measurement of central venous pressure gives an accurate picture of the changing hydration status of the animal. A high central venous pressure can indicate over administration of fluid, occlusion of the catheter or right ventricular heart failure. A low central venous pressure may indicate reduced blood volume. *Changes* in central venous pressure are more important than absolute values: these changes give an indication of the hydration status of the animal and the response to treatment.

3

Which fluid and why?

Key points

- Blood products, colloids and crystalloids are the three main fluid types used in veterinary practice
- Blood transfusion requires a suitable donor and checks for compatibility
- The aim is to replace 'like with like' by choosing appropriate fluids for the condition and the expected or actual water/electrolyte losses occurring in the patient
- Potassium levels should ideally be monitored and any disturbances treated as necessary

The aim of fluid therapy is to replace losses and maintain fluid and electrolyte balance in the body, thus allowing for normal cell and organ function. A number of commercially available fluids are suitable for this purpose, and will be discussed in this chapter.

To understand where a fluid is going after it leaves the intravenous catheter, a basic knowledge of fluid distribution in the body is required (see Ch. 1). It is important to remember that the fluid compartments in the body exchange fluid to compensate for losses: thus fluid lost initially from one compartment inevitably results in a loss from all compartments.

Classification of fluids

The fluids used in intravenous fluid therapy are generally classified into the following three groups:

1. Whole blood and blood products
2. Colloids
3. Crystalloids.

Whole blood and blood products

Whole blood is used in cases of:

- Severe haemorrhage
- Severe anemia

- Specific problems (e.g. Von Willebrand's disease) where it is necessary to provide platelets or clotting factors.

Blood collection

Blood is collected from the donor animal using a blood collection bag containing an anticoagulant: citrate phosphate dextrose (CPD) is commonly used. The blood donor must be clinically healthy and have a normal packed cell volume. Dogs should weigh a minimum of 25 kg; cats should not be obese and should test FeLV, FIV and FIA negative.

It is a legal requirement in the UK that blood may only be taken from an animal for a specific patient: blood cannot be taken from a donor and then stored for use on any patient in the future. Some large establishments keep donor dogs on site but this is impractical in most practice situations due to economic and space restrictions. The donor is often a pet belonging to a member of staff or a willing client and can be called upon when needed. If blood is taken from a donor animal for a specific patient but is then *not* used (e.g. if the animal dies) or if not all the donor blood is used, surplus blood can be stored. Whole blood can be stored between 1–6°C for up to three weeks.

Blood is usually collected from dogs using a standard blood collection bag (Fig. 3.1). One unit (400 mL) can be collected safely from the donor. If the primary purpose of the transfusion is administration of red cells, sight hounds (e.g. Greyhounds) that have a naturally high packed cell volume are preferred as donors. The donor dog does not usually require sedation. Blood is collected from the jugular vein and local anaesthetic may be infiltrated into the skin before venepuncture. During collection, the dog is kept in a comfortable position – sitting, standing or sternal recumbency – and the vein is raised. The collection needle, which is pre-attached to the blood collection bag by the manufacturer, is placed into the vein and held firmly during collection. The bag is held below the donor and agitated gently during collection to mix the blood with the anticoagulant. Collection is continued until the bag is full: weighing the bag or identifying when it is turgid with blood assesses fullness (Fig. 3.2). After the needle has been removed from the vein, a firm neck bandage is kept in place for two hours to avoid the formation of a haematoma.

Blood collection from cats is also from the jugular vein and is collected into a large syringe. Donor cats may require sedation although this should be avoided unless absolutely necessary. Up to 50 mL can be collected from a large healthy cat. 1 mL of anticoagulant is drawn into the syringe for every 9 mL of blood to be collected. The cat is restrained in a sitting position or upside down in the handler's lap. The blood is collected with a large (20 G) needle using good venepuncture technique.

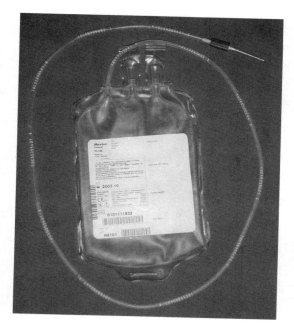

Figure 3.1 Blood collection bag before use. It contains anticoagulant and has a needle attached.

Blood grouping

In dogs, there are eight isoantibody (blood grouping) systems, given the numbers 1–8. The only one that has any real clinical importance is DEA (dog erythrocyte antigen) 1. Whilst all of the dog blood groups can potentially stimulate transfusion reactions, DEA 1 will cause the most severe reaction. Dogs can be blood typed and dogs that are DEA 1 positive should be avoided as donors.

In cats, the blood groups are much simpler. There are basically three groups: A, B and AB. Cats should be cross-matched or blood typed before any transfusion, since there is a significant risk of a clinically important transfusion reaction.

Although transfusion reactions rarely occur in dogs that have not been transfused before, the risk of a reaction occurring increases with each transfusion that is given. This means that, ideally, donor and recipient dogs should be blood typed and dogs or cats that have been transfused previously should be cross-matched before subsequent transfusions. Blood typing is more accurate than cross-matching since blood typing

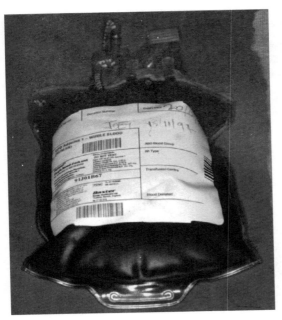

Figure 3.2 Full blood collection bag. The bag appears turgid and can be weighed to assess fullness.

looks for particular antigens on the surface of the red blood cell. Commercial blood testing kits are available for use in general veterinary practice. Where these kits are not available, cross-matching the donor and recipient blood helps to avoid transfusion reactions.

Cross-matching helps to avoid any incompatibility reactions. It involves taking a blood sample from the donor and recipient and testing to determine cross-reactions between plasma and red blood cells. This predicts the likelihood of an immediate transfusion reaction happening – it does not predict future antibody reactions.

Preferably, a full cross-match should be performed. An EDTA blood sample from the donor and the recipient is centrifuged at 3000 rpm for 10 minutes and the supernatant removed. The erythrocytes are resuspended in saline and this is centrifuged again at 3000 rpm for 10 minutes. The supernatant is removed and the erythrocytes are resuspended again in saline to make a 3–5% solution. A *major cross-match* will assess the effect that recipient serum antibodies will have on donor cells. It is performed by mixing two drops of donor red cell suspension with one or two drops of recipient plasma in a test tube. A positive result is

---

Box 3.1   Simple blood compatibility test

Cross-matching can be performed in general veterinary practice. A simple compatibility test can be performed on blood:

- Place two drops of donor blood in EDTA into 1 mL of saline and add two drops of patient serum.
- Centrifuge at a low speed for 15–30 seconds.
- Flick the tube to resuspend.
- If signs of agglutination are present this suggests incompatibility.
- This test does not test for haemolysis.

---

indicated by haemolysis or agglutination. A *minor cross-match* will assess the effect that donor serum will have on recipient cells. It is performed by mixing two drops of recipient red cell suspension with one or two drops of donor plasma in a test tube. Incubate the test tube at 37°C for 60 minutes. Haemolysis or agglutination indicates a positive result.

Administration of blood

Blood is administered to the recipient through a blood giving set with filter (Fig. 3.3). The purpose of the filter is to remove any clots and prevent them from entering the recipient's circulation. The flow rate of the blood administration set must be noted in calculating the rate of infusion of blood. Blood should be carefully warmed to 37°C prior to administration – overheating will result in agglutination and protein breakdown.

Blood is administered at an initial rate of 0.25 mL/kg/hour for the first 15 minutes. Constant monitoring of the recipient during this time enables observation of any potential transfusion reaction. The rate is then increased to 20 mL/kg/hour. The total volume of blood is administered over 2–4 hours.

Giving an animal blood does involve some practical problems. If clotting factors and platelets are to be supplied, the blood must be given immediately it is taken from the donor: it cannot be stored. Incompatibility reactions are most likely in the first hour following transfusion and the patient must be monitored closely. There are numerous signs that indicate a transfusion reaction (Box 3.2) and these can vary from very mild to serious life-threatening situations. If the patient is showing any abnormal clinical signs the veterinary surgeon should be

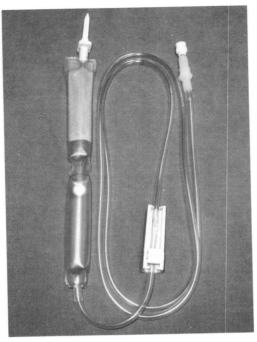

Figure 3.3 A blood giving set incorporating a filter to remove clots.

Box 3.2   Clinical signs associated with blood transfusion reactions

- Urticaria
- Hypersalivation
- Muscle tremors
- Tachycardia
- Vomiting/nausea
- Restlessness
- Jaundice
- Dyspnoea
- Haemoglobinuria
- Pyrexia
- Facial oedema
- Tachypnoea
- Convulsions

informed immediately and the transfusion stopped. The usual treatment of a blood transfusion reaction is to administer crystalloid fluids, antihistamines, antibiotics and corticosteroids.

Oxyglobin™

Oxyglobin™ (Fig. 3.4) is a plasma volume expander containing haemoglobin that improves oxygen delivery by increasing the oxygen content of the blood and expanding vascular volume. It is currently only licensed for use in dogs and is indicated in cases of severe anemia. The main advantages in using Oxyglobin™ rather than whole blood is that no blood typing or cross-matching is necessary since a transfusion reaction is unlikely. There is no need for a donor animal – thus saving time. However the cost of Oxyglobin™ currently prohibits regular use of the product.

Side effects can be seen. A transient red-brown discolouration of patient's urine, a yellow-red discolouration of skin, mucous membranes

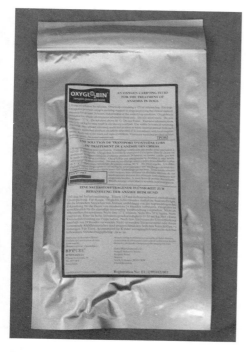

Figure 3.4 Oxyglobin™ – a plasma expander containing haemoglobin – is an alternative to blood tranfusion.

and sclera and yellow/orange/red spots on skin may be noted. These minor side effects usually last for 3–5 days.

Oxyglobin™ is warmed to 37°C prior to use and is administered via a standard giving set and intravenous catheter. It must not be administered in conjunction with any other fluids. The recommended dose is 30 mL/kg intravenously at a rate of up to 10 mL/kg/hour.

Colloids

Colloids are a group of fluids containing large molecules designed to remain in the intravenous space longer than crystalloid fluids. This means that colloids are able to expand and maintain the vascular volume more effectively. Their osmotic potential is so great that colloids draw fluid out of the interstitial and intracellular spaces into the plasma, hence colloids are commonly termed *plasma expanders*.

Colloids are used in cases of shock where cardiovascular function needs to be improved rapidly:

• Haemorrhage
• Shock
• Severe dehydration.

Following haemorrhage, colloids are sometimes administered rather than blood because obtaining a blood donor is not always easy and they avoid the possibility of a blood transfusion reaction if cross-matching is not possible or practical.

Dextrans

These are artificial colloids with a high molecular weight. They are not available on the veterinary market in the UK but are available in the USA.

Gelatins

Gelatins are straw coloured, isotonic colloid solutions. The two trade names in common use in the UK are Haemaccel™ and Gelofusin™. Gelatins should be stored at room temperature. They are administered through a standard fluid administration set and intravenous catheter. The patient does not require cross-matching before administration and gelatins must not be administered with whole blood.

Plasma

Plasma is also considered in this fluid category. Whole blood can be separated, e.g. by centrifugation, into plasma and packed red cells.

However, facilities for this are rarely available in general veterinary practice. When possible, it does allow the patient to receive specific treatment with plasma proteins, whilst minimising the risk of a cross-reaction. See also Oxyglobin™ above.

Crystalloids

Crystalloids are a group of sodium-based electrolyte fluids. They enter the extracellular fluid (ECF) and from there equilibriate with other fluid compartments in the body to restore fluid balance. The most commonly used crystalloids are similar to plasma water in composition. In patients where renal function is normal, crystalloids will be excreted in the urine.

Hartmann's (lactated Ringer's) solution

Hartmann's contains electrolytes in very similar concentrations to those in the extracellular fluid (ECF). Sodium (Na^+), potassium (K^+), calcium (Ca^{++}), chloride (Cl^-) and lactate are present.

Hartmann's is indicated in many cases of fluid and electrolyte losses. The lactate present is metabolised to bicarbonate, and this is used in the body to overcome situations of metabolic acidosis, which occur in many clinical conditions.

0.9% sodium chloride (saline)

This solution contains sodium (Na^+) and chloride (Cl^-), but no potassium (K^+). 0.9% sodium chloride is indicated in fluid and electrolyte losses, particularly when plasma potassium levels are increased due to underlying disease and additional administration of potassium must be avoided during fluid therapy.

5% dextrose

5% dextrose, also referred to as 5% glucose, is basically water with a small amount (50 mg/mL) of glucose added in order to make it isotonic, thus enabling it to be administered intravenously. This solution contains no electrolytes so provides the body with water and a very small amount of glucose. 5% dextrose is indicated in situations of primary water loss, where the animal is unable to take in oral fluids, and in cases of hypoglycaemia. The amount of glucose present is too little to make a significant contribution to the energy intake of the animal.

0.18% sodium chloride and 4% glucose (glucose-saline)

Glucose-saline is mainly water but also has a small amount of sodium and chloride to replace daily urinary losses in the normal animal. It is used in cases of primary water loss and occasionally as a maintenance fluid, although in the latter case potassium should be added to the drip bag.

Ringer's solution

Ringer's solution contains mainly sodium, chloride and some potassium. It is indicated in water and electrolyte loss when there is also some potassium deficit. It is mainly used in cases of pyometra when severe vomiting is present. Vomiting leads to substantial losses of hydrogen and chloride which in turn produces an excess of sodium. The kidneys try to compensate for the sodium excess, which can give rise to hypokalaemia.

Darrow's solution

This solution contains sodium, chloride, and potassium in higher concentrations than Ringer's or Hartmann's. Darrow's solution is mainly indicated in cases of metabolic acidosis with potassium deficiency, e.g. persistent diarrhoea.

Hypertonic saline (7.8% or 9% sodium chloride)

Hypertonic saline is under-used in small animal intravenous fluid therapy, but is more widely accepted in large animal fluid therapy (see Ch. 8). When this type of sodium chloride is administered intravenously, its high osmotic potential causes fluid from the intracellular space to move into the vascular space. This causes a sudden rapid increase in circulating volume that is needed in cases of severe hypovolaemia. Hypertonic saline is therefore indicated in situations such as: gastric dilation and

Table 3.1 Replacement fluid constituents for commonly used products

Fluid	Na^+ (mmol/L)	Cl^- (mmol/L)	K^+ (mmol/L)	Ca^{++} (mmol/L)	Others
0.9% sodium chloride	154	154	–	–	–
Hartmann's solution	131	111	5	2	Lactate
Ringer's solution	147	156	4	2.5	–
5% dextrose	–	–	–	–	5% dextrose
0.18% NaCl & 4% dextrose	30	30	–	–	4% dextrose
Darrow's solution	121	103	35	–	Lactate
Haemaccel	145	150	5	3	Gelatins
Hypertonic saline	855	855	–	–	–
Normal plasma	145	100	5	–	Lactate

volvulus (GDV), equine colic, severe haemorrhage. Typically, a 7.8% solution of hypertonic saline is administered intravenously at a rate of 4–5 mL/kg.

Potassium supplementation

Potassium may be added to a crystalloid fluid in cases of hypokalaemia. However, potassium supplementation is not often performed in general practice since it should only be carried out when blood potassium levels can be measured, and many practices are unable to do this using in-house blood analysers.

Hypokalaemia becomes important when plasma levels fall below 3.5 mmol/L. Patient potassium levels should be measured and potassium supplementation administered accordingly in 'at risk' patients (Box 3.3). Recommended supplementation doses are shown in Table 3.2. Potassium supplementation doses of 0.5 mmol/L/kg/hour should not be exceeded due to risks of hyperkalaemia and cardiotoxicity.

If potassium is added to a bag of crystalloid fluid it must be mixed thoroughly by inverting the bag of fluid several times. The fluid bag must then be labelled to indicate that potassium has been added.

Box 3.3   Common causes and signs of hypokalaemia

Causes	Signs
Vomiting	Weakness
Diarrhoea	Lethargy
Renal disease	Anorexia
Anorexia	Ileus
Diet low in potassium	
Aggressive diuretic therapy	

Table 3.2   Potassium replacement doses in hypokalaemia

Serum potassium (mmol/L)	Potassium chloride added to fluids (mmol/L)
3.6–5.0	20
3.1–3.5	30
2.6–3.0	40
2.1–2.5	60
<2.0	80

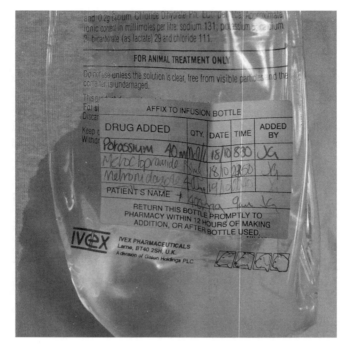

and 0.2g Calcium Chloride Dihydrate Ph. Eur. per litre. Approximate ionic content in millimoles per litre: sodium 131; potassium; calcium ; bicarbonate (as lactate) 29 and chloride 111.

FOR ANIMAL TREATMENT ONLY

Do not use unless the solution is clear, free from visible particles and the container is undamaged.

AFFIX TO INFUSION BOTTLE

DRUG ADDED	QTY.	DATE	TIME	ADDED BY
Potassium 40 mmol		18/10	830	JG
Metoclopramide		18/10	2260	JG
Metronidazole		19/10		

PATIENT'S NAME

RETURN THIS BOTTLE PROMPTLY TO PHARMACY WITHIN 12 HOURS OF MAKING ADDITION, OR AFTER BOTTLE USED.

IVEX PHARMACEUTICALS
Larne, BT40 2SH, U.K.
A division of Galen Holdings PLC

Figure 3.5 It is important that potassium and other additives are noted clearly on infusion bags and in the patient's clinical record.

Clinical situations requiring fluid therapy

When presented with a clinical case, a decision must be made as to which fluid to use to treat the animal's condition. Generally we try to 'replace like with like'. This simply means that where blood is lost, replace the deficit with blood; where water is lost, replace with water; and where water and electrolytes are lost, replace water and electrolytes.

Blood loss

Blood loss reduces the circulating volume and perfusion, and therefore reduces the oxygen carrying capacity of blood. A low packed cell volume (PCV) indicates this. In severe blood loss oxygenation of the tissues is significantly compromised. Generally, if the PCV falls below 20% then a blood transfusion is necessary. During surgery, if the patient loses more than 18 mL/kg of blood then a blood transfusion is also indicated. Anemia and bleeding disorders can be an indication for blood to

Table 3.3 Indications for different replacement fluids

Fluid	Indications for use
0.9% sodium chloride	Alkalosis, vomiting, urinary obstruction, hepatic disease
Hartmann's solution	Diarrhoea, acidosis, endocrine disease
Ringer's solution	Pyometra, severe vomiting
5% dextrose	Primary water loss, hypoglycaemia
0.18% NaCl & 4% dextrose	Maintenance requirements, hypoglycaemia
Darrow's solution	Severe diarrhoea
Haemaccel	Blood loss
Hypertonic saline	Severe haemorrhage, hypovolaemia
Blood	Haemorrhage

be given. Many animals with chronic anemia, however, will tolerate a low PCV without clinical signs.

For severe blood loss, using the 'like for like' rule, blood is the first choice of replacement fluid. If blood is unavailable, the second fluid choice is a colloid; this will expand the vascular space. If there is no colloid, then a crystalloid can be given. Hartmann's is most similar in composition to plasma. Blood volume needs to be replaced and whilst this is being carried out it is necessary to monitor PCV to ensure this remains at a sufficient level for oxygen requirements.

A packed cell volume of 20–25% is considered a minimum level in acutely affected animals (chronic cases will tolerate lower PCVs).

Primary water loss

This is loss of water with little or no loss of electrolytes. In this situation, water only needs to be replaced. Common conditions causing this include fractured jaw, panting, neglect by owners and unconsciousness. Crystalloids are the fluids of choice: 5% dextrose or 0.18% sodium chloride and 4% glucose are used.

Loss of water and electrolytes

This occurs as a result of conditions producing clinical signs such as vomiting and diarrhoea. A crystalloid containing both water and electrolytes must be used to replace the deficit. An important consideration in deciding which crystalloid to use is whether potassium is being lost or is accumulating in the body. This ion is important for normal metabolism and plasma potassium concentration must remain stable within narrow limits in order for body cells to function normally.

Table 3.4 Common clinical conditions and suggested fluids

Condition and consequences	Need to supply	Fluid of choice	Comments
Diarrhoea • Loss of water and electrolytes • Loss of K^+ through GI tract • Metabolic acidosis	• Water and electrolytes • K^+ • Bicarbonate/lactate	Hartmann's solution	
Severe blood loss • e.g. during surgery	• Red blood cells and plasma	Whole blood	
Vomiting • Loss of water and electrolytes • Metabolic alkalosis	• Water and electrolytes	0.9% NaCl	If vomiting progresses, K^+ will be lost and must be replaced: Hartmann's or Ringer's can be given
Pyometra A complicated situation with many disease processes present • Loss of K^+ since animal may be vomiting, anorexic; patient often has a vaginal discharge • If patient is shocked, will become acidotic • If patient is vomiting profusely, will become alkalotic • Patients with pyometra are *usually* considered acidotic	• Water and electrolytes • K^+ • Correct acidosis	Hartmann's solution	
Anorexia • Primary water loss	• Water	0.18% NaCl + 4% dextrose	If prolonged, anorexia leads to loss of K^+ so Hartmann's is indicated
Urinary tract obstruction (cats) • Hyperkalaemia	• Water and electrolytes	0.9% NaCl	Build up of K^+ is more life threatening than metabolic acidosis, so ensure fluids administered do not contain K^+

In the healthy animal, potassium is lost slowly in urine and is obtained through food. Any disease affecting either of these two functions will alter potassium levels in the body, e.g. excessive losses in urine lead to potassium depletion; urinary tract obstruction leads to an accumulation of potassium since it is not excreted; starved animals are unable to obtain potassium in food, so depletion occurs.

> In conditions of potential potassium depletion, a crystalloid containing potassium and other electrolytes to replace losses is required. In conditions of potential potassium accumulation, then crystalloids containing potassium must be avoided.

The final consideration when selecting a fluid is any change in the animal's acid–base balance (see also Ch. 4). In situations of metabolic acidosis, bicarbonate ions are needed – this is achieved by supplying lactate (contained in Hartmann's solution), which is metabolised by the body into bicarbonate. Sodium bicarbonate solution is also available to add to crystalloid fluids. In situations of metabolic alkalosis, bicarbonate should not be given to the animal and crystalloid fluids containing lactate should be avoided.

Hartmann's solution and whole blood must not be administered via the same catheter at the same time because the calcium in Hartmann's solution causes blood to clot. Administration to the same patient at the same time using separate i.v. catheters is however permissible, and this is also true for other calcium-containing fluid therapy products.

Table 3.4 outlines the fluid therapy requirements for some of the commonest conditions encountered in general veterinary practice.

4

Acid–base balance

> **Key points**
>
> - Blood pH is regulated within very close limits
> - Abnormalities in pH are known as acid–base imbalances and can have serious effects
> - Many common diseases may cause acid–base imbalances
> - Accurate assessment of acid–base status requires blood gas analysis

Body fluids must be maintained at a certain pH for normal body processes to work. The pH is a measurement of the concentration of hydrogen ions and we can refer to the acidity or alkalinity of a solution. A neutral solution at 25°C has a pH of 7; a pH below 7 indicates an acidic solution; a pH above 7 indicates an alkaline solution. For normal cell metabolism the body needs to maintain its pH within a narrow range. The normal pH of blood is 7.35–7.45. When blood pH falls below 7.35, a state of *acidosis* exists. When blood pH rises to above 7.45, a state of *alkalosis* exists. If the pH moves outside the normal range this becomes a serious problem: cells (and therefore tissues and organs) do not function correctly, eventually leading to death.

pH control

There are numerous conditions and processes that may occur in an animal which could cause either acidosis or alkalosis. If there were no compensating mechanisms within the body, then the pH would quickly change and the animal's life would be at risk.

A change in blood pH seems almost inevitable since the body, during normal metabolism, is constantly producing hydrogen ions. The breakdown of nutrients in digestion results in the production of acids. There are three ways in which the body keeps hydrogen ions at a constant level, therefore controlling pH: through actions of the renal system, the respiratory system and by using buffers.

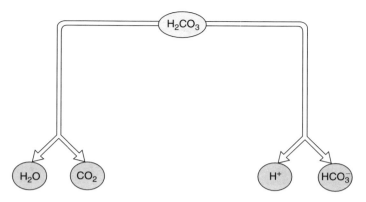

Figure 4.1 In the normal animal, the 'scales' are balanced by equal amounts of each chemical.

Renal system

The kidney nephrons can excrete or retain bicarbonate ions in response to the acid–base balance of the body. Renal function is of great importance to the maintenance of normal pH. If a medical condition or disease impairs the renal system then a change in body pH is likely.

Respiratory system

The respiratory system controls the levels of carbon dioxide (CO_2) in the body. In order to understand how this affects pH, a chemical reaction named the Henderson–Hasselbalch equation needs to be considered:

$$H_2O + CO_2 \rightleftharpoons H_2CO_3 \rightleftharpoons H^+ + HCO_3^-$$

Carbonic   Hydrogen   Bicarbonate
acid   ion

This chemical equation shows water and carbon dioxide reacting to produce carbonic acid. The carbonic acid can breakdown into water and carbon dioxide again or into hydrogen ion and bicarbonate, i.e. the chemical reactions are *reversible*, with each of the chemicals existing *in equilibrium*. We can imagine this chemical equation as a pair of scales (Fig. 4.1). If carbon dioxide and water are lost, the scales will move (Fig. 4.2).

Carbon dioxide is expired during normal respiration and blood pH is kept constant. However, abnormalities in respiration can cause a change in pH of the blood. If the respiratory rate and volume decrease, carbon dioxide accumulates, more hydrogen ions are produced (see equation), the pH lowers and the animal becomes *acidotic*. If the respiratory rate

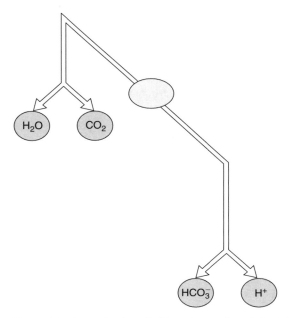

Figure 4.2 Loss of carbon dioxide and water disrupts the balance and results in a temporary increase of bicarbonate and hydrogen ions, before equilibrium is re-established.

increases, carbon dioxide is depleted, less hydrogen ions are produced, the pH rises and the animal becomes *alkalotic*.

> • If hydrogen ion concentration falls, blood pH rises and the animal becomes alkalotic.
> • If hydrogen ion concentration increases, blood pH falls and the animal becomes acidotic.

Buffers

A buffer is a substance to which hydrogen ions will attach or can be detached from, therefore changing the amount of hydrogen ions in circulation. Buffers can be likened to a sponge: a buffer can attract hydrogen ions as a sponge attracts water. Similarly, hydrogen ions can be detached from a buffer as a sponge is squeezed of water. Bicarbonate, phosphate, haemoglobin and plasma proteins are all important buffers in the body, compensating for small changes in pH.

Fluid therapy and acid–base balance

If any of the in-built mechanisms to keep a constant pH in the body are impaired, the animal will suffer an acid–base disturbance. Fluid therapy can help correct an acid–base balance disturbance, e.g. by providing lactate which is metabolised into bicarbonate. This is needed in acidosis, when the body has an increase in hydrogen ions.

Alternatively, if the body has an excess of bicarbonate ions, as in alkalosis, it is important *not* to administer a fluid containing lactate. Extra bicarbonate should not be added to an animal already suffering from alkalosis. Fluid therapy is still helpful as the fluid dilutes the imbalance. It also encourages renal function, which aids restoration of normal pH by means of kidney regulation mechanisms.

Common abnormalities of acid–base balance

Although the body has built-in mechanisms to overcome the inevitable constant small changes in acid–base, there are occasions when the animal has a medical condition which the body's regulatory mechanisms cannot cope with. See Box 4.1.

Metabolic acidosis

Metabolic acidosis arises when acid metabolites are retained in the body and an accumulation of hydrogen ions occurs. For example, if

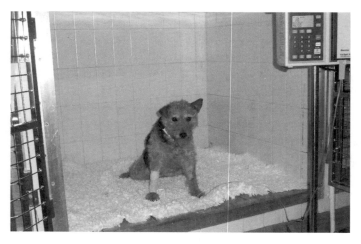

Figure 4.3 Fluid therapy is important in the treatment of acid–base imbalances.

> # Box 4.1 Common causes of acid–base disturbances
>
> **Metabolic acidosis**
> - Renal failure
> - Ruptured bladder
> - Urethral obstruction
> - Lower urinary tract disease
> - Shock
>
> **Metabolic alkalosis**
> - Vomiting
> - Overadministration of bicarbonate, e.g. during fluid therapy
>
> **Respiratory acidosis**
> - Acute respiratory obstruction or failure
> - Severe lung disease
> - Faulty anaesthetic equipment
> - Respiratory depression
>
> **Respiratory alkalosis**
> - Hyperventilation, e.g. pain

the kidneys become impaired, due to trauma or disease, then they may be unable to excrete hydrogen ions. A build up occurs and the animal becomes acidotic. Ruptured bladder (e.g. following a road traffic accident) or a blocked urethra in lower urinary tract disease are common conditions which create this effect.

Metabolic acidosis is generally common in the ill or shocked animal. In these cases, poor tissue perfusion results in the production of lactic acid during cell metabolism, leading to hydrogen ion accumulation.

Metabolic alkalosis

Metabolic alkalosis arises when hydrogen ions are lost from the body in abnormal quantities. Vomiting depletes hydrogen ions from the body since the gastric mucosa normally secretes hydrogen ions that are subsequently absorbed by the body. During vomiting, these hydrogen ions are expelled from the body, creating a metabolic alkalosis.

Respiratory acidosis

Respiratory acidosis is an acute problem and occurs when carbon dioxide accumulates in the body. The carbon dioxide reacts with water to form carbonic acid; carbonic acid then breaks down to release hydrogen ions, causing acidosis. When an animal experiences respiratory obstruction or depression, respiratory function is impaired and carbon dioxide accumulates. Alternatively, an animal might inspire an excess of carbon dioxide from faulty anaesthetic equipment. Both situations lead to respiratory acidosis.

Respiratory alkalosis

Respiratory alkalosis arises due to an excessive loss of carbon dioxide from the body. This may be as a result of hyperventilation due to apprehension, pain or fear. Respiratory alkalosis is seen less frequently than acidosis. It is uncommon to breathe so rapidly that a significant loss of carbon dioxide occurs.

Measurement of acid–base balance

Acid–base balance is commonly assessed by blood gas analysis. An arterial blood sample is collected, without contamination by air, into a heparinised syringe. A blood gas analyser machine measures the pH and the amount of bicarbonate in the blood. Many analyser machines also measure the 'base excess', which quantifies the degree of pH imbalance and how much bicarbonate the body needs to correct the problem. Many veterinary practices do not have a blood gas analyser machine available for use, so direct measurement of acid–base balance is not possible.

5

Calculating fluid requirements and flow rates

Key points

- Maintenance fluid requirements are estimated at 50 mL/kg/24 hours
- Deficit fluid requirements are calculated according to accepted estimations of losses
- Drip rates are calculated from giving set drip factors
- Calculation of fluid requirements avoids dangerous under or overadministration of fluid therapy

---

To calculate the amount of fluid to administer to an animal, a step-by-step approach should be followed:

1. Calculate how much fluid is needed to replace fluid that has been lost. This may be estimated by clinical examination of the patient *or* laboratory tests *or* inferred from the animal's history. This fluid to replace losses is termed the *deficit* (see Ch. 2).
2. Calculate how much fluid the animal would normally take in over the period of time it will be kept on intravenous fluids – this is the normal *maintenance*. This can be estimated as 50 mL/kg/24hours.
3. Add together deficit and maintenance to give the *total fluid requirement*.

Worked examples for fluid replacement calculations

Example 1

A 10 kg dog is 5% dehydrated. Calculate its fluid requirement for the next 24 hour period.

---

1. *Deficit:* 5% dehydrated = $5 \div 100 \times 10\,kg = 0.5\,kg$
   We know that 1 kg = 1 L, therefore 0.5 kg = 0.5 L
   There are 1000 mL in 1 L, so 0.5 L = 500 mL

> Deficit = 500 mL

2. *Maintenance:* 50 mL/kg/24 hours
   For this patient: 50 mL × 10 kg × 24 hours = 500 mL

> Maintenance = 500 mL over 24 hours

3. *Total fluid requirement = deficit + maintenance*
   500 mL + 500 mL = 1000 mL

> Total required = 1000 mL = 1 L over 24 hours

Example 2

A 4 kg cat had a PCV of 37%. It became severely dehydrated and PCV is now 49%. Calculate the fluid needed for the next 24 hour period.

---

1. *Deficit:* this is an increase in PCV of 12%
   For each 1% increase in PCV, we know there is a fluid loss of approximately 10 mL/kg.
   So for this cat: 12% × 10 mL × 4 kg = 480 mL

> Deficit = 480 mL

2. *Maintenance:* 50 mL/kg/24 hours
   For this patient: 50 mL × 4 kg = 200 mL/24 hours

> Maintenance = 200 mL

3. *Total fluid requirement = deficit + maintenance*
   480 mL + 200 mL = 680 mL

> Total required = 680 mL over 24 hours

Example 3

A 20 kg dog requires fluid at twice maintenance. Calculate its fluid requirement over 24 hours.

1. *Maintenance*: 50 mL/kg/24 hours
   Twice maintenance = 2 × 50 mL/kg/24 hours
   For this patient: 2 × 50 mL × 20 kg = 2000 mL/24 hours

The requirement is 2000 mL or 2 L over 24 hours.

Calculation of drip rate

Having calculated how much fluid the animal requires over a 24 hour period, the next step is to work out how fast to set the drip flowing through the giving set. On the packaging of giving sets the drip factor, also known as the giving set rate, is shown. The drip factor is the number of drops in 1 mL. A giving set commonly has a drip factor of 15 or 20. This means it delivers 15 or 20 drops per 1 mL of fluid.

A step-by-step guide can be used to calculate the drip rate:

1. Determine the fluid deficit in mL.
2. Determine the 24 hour maintenance required in mL.
3. Determine the amount of fluid in mL per hour (this is deficit plus maintenance divided by 24).
4. Determine the amount of fluid in mL per minute (this is the amount of fluid per hour divided by 60).
5. Determine the amount of fluid in drops per minute (this is the mL per minute multiplied by the drip factor).
6. Determine 1 drop every x seconds by dividing 60 with the number of drops per minute.

Example 4

A 10 kg dog requires 500 mL of fluid to be administered over the next 24 hours to replace losses, and 500 mL of fluid for maintenance. The giving set delivers 20 drops per mL. Calculate the drip rate.

1. Fluid deficit in mL = 500 mL
2. Maintenance in mL = 500 mL
3. Calculate total amount of fluid per hour over 24 hours:
   500 mL + 500 mL = 1000 mL
   Divide this by 24 hours: 1000 mL/24 = 41.6 mL/hour

4. Calculate mL per minute: 41.6 mL/hour ÷ 60 = 0.69 mL/minute
5. Calculate drops per minute: 0.69 mL/minute × drip factor of 20 = 13.88 drops/minute
6. Calculate 1 drop every x seconds: 60 ÷ 13.88 drops/minute = 4.3

> Answer: 1 drop should be received every 4 seconds.

The nurse should set the giving set, infusion pump or syringe driver to deliver one drop every four seconds to the patient.

Clinical case questions and worked answers

Case 1

A 5 kg German Shepherd puppy has acute vomiting and diarrhoea. He has vomited 10 times and passed 5 fluid motions. What is his fluid requirement over the next 24 hours? The fluid will be administered via a burette which has a drip factor of 60. What is the drip rate?

1. *Deficit*: This is worked out from known vomiting and diarrhoea figures:
   4 mL × 5 kg × 10 vomits = 200 mL
   4 mL × 5 kg × 5 diarrhoea = 100 mL
   Total deficit = 200 + 100 = 300 mL
2. *Maintenance*: 50 mL/kg/24 hours
   For this patient: 50 mL × 5 kg = 250 mL over 24 hours
   Maintenance = 250 mL
3. Fluid per hour = deficit + maintenance/24 hours
   300 mL + 250 mL = 550 mL
   550 mL ÷ 24 hours = 22.9 mL/hour
4. Calculate mL per minute: 22.9 mL/hour ÷ 60 = 0.38 mL/minute
5. Calculate drops per minute: 0.38 × drip factor of 60 = 22.8 drops/minute
6. Calculate 1 drop to be given every x seconds: 60 ÷ 22.8 drops/minute = 2.63 seconds
   Practically, this is rounded up to 1 drop to be given every 3 seconds

> Answer: 24-hour fluid requirement for this case is 550 mL.
> Give 1 drop every 3 seconds to achieve this.

Case 2

A 25 kg dog has suffered heat stroke and is to be given fluids at twice the rate of maintenance over 24 hours. What is the dog's fluid requirement? The drip factor is 20. Calculate the drip rate.

1. *Maintenance*: 50 mL/kg/24 hours
   For this patient: 50 mL × 25 kg = 1250 mL/24 hours
   Twice this patient's maintenance: 1250 mL × 2 = 2500 mL/24 hours
2. Fluid per hour: 2500 mL ÷ 24 hours = 104.1 mL/hour
3. mL per minute: 104.1 mL/hour ÷ 60 = 1.73 mL/minute
4. Drops per minute: 1.73 mL/minute × drip factor of 20 = 34.7 drops/minute
5. Calculate 1 drop every x seconds: 60 ÷ 34.7 drops/minute = 1.7 seconds
   Practically, this is rounded up to 1 drop to be given every 2 seconds

Answer: Maintenance requirement is 2500 mL (2.5 L) over 24 hours. Give 1 drop every 2 seconds to achieve this.

Case 3

A 3 kg cat has just had surgery. She is to receive 1.5 times total daily maintenance fluids, administered via a burette, over the next 8 hours. The burette drip factor is 60. Calculate the amount of fluid and the drip rate.

1. *Maintenance*: 50 mL/kg/24 hours
   For this patient: 50 mL × 3 kg = 150 mL
   1.5 × maintenance: 1.5 × 150 mL = 225 mL
2. 225 mL is to be given over 8 hours
   This means: 225 mL ÷ 8 = 28.1 mL/hour
3. Calculate mL/minute: 28.1 mL/hour ÷ 60 = 0.46 mL/minute
4. Calculate drops/minute: 0.46 mL/minute × drip factor 60 = 28.1 drops/minute
5. Calculate 1 drop every x seconds: 60 ÷ 28.1 drops/minute = 2.1 seconds
   Practically, this is rounded up to 1 drop to be given every 2 seconds

Answer: Amount of fluid required is 225 mL. Give 1 drop every 2 seconds over 8 hours.

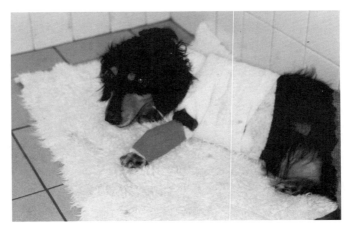

Figure 5.1   Correct i.v. fluid therapy can be vital in postoperative patients. Requirements should always be assessed by the calculation methods described in this chapter, rather than by 'guesswork'.

Acute fluid loss

In some situations of severe or acute deficit, fluid therapy is tailored to restore the vascular volume quickly and then restore the total body water more slowly. For example, 25% of the deficit may be given rapidly over the first hour, and then the remainder more slowly over the following 23 hours. Often, a plasma expander (colloid, see Ch. 3) is used to replace the first part of the deficit.

Case 4

A 20 kg dog is 10% dehydrated. It is desired to replace 25% of the deficit in the first hour of fluid therapy, and the remainder of the requirement over the next 23 hours. Work out the total fluid requirement and the volume to be given in the first hour.

---

1. *Deficit*: 10% of 20 kg = 2 kg = 2 L
2. *Maintenance*: 50 mL/kg/24 hours
   For this patient: 50 mL × 20 kg = 1 L over 24 hours
3. *Total fluid requirement*: 2 L + 1 L = 3 L
4. 25% of total *deficit*: deficit = 2 L therefore 25% of 2 L = 0.5 L = 500 mL

Answer: Total fluid requirement = 3 L
Volume to be given in the first hour = 500 mL
Give the remainder of the deficit plus maintenance over the next 23 hours.

6

Administration of fluid therapy

Key points

- The commonest and most useful route for fluid administration is the intravenous one
- Intraosseous, subcutaneous and intraperitoneal are also used in the hospital situation
- Catheters must be placed with care and using good technique if they are to function well
- A range of devices and equipment is available to facilitate intravenous fluid administration

A number of different routes can be used for the administration of fluid therapy in animals. These will be discussed in this chapter, and practical guidelines given. Common abbreviations that are used in textbooks and journals for the various fluid therapy routes are listed in Table 6.1.

Methods of fluid administration

Table 6.2 and the following text outlines the advantages and disadvantages of the different routes of fluid administration.

Table 6.1 Abbreviations to describe routes of administration

Routes for fluid administration	Abbreviations in common use
Oral	*Per os*; p.o.
Subcutaneous	s.c.; s/c; S/C; S/Q
Intraperitoneal	i.p.; i/p; I/P
Rectal	None commonly used
Intraosseous	i.o.; i/o; I/O
Intravenous	i.v.; i/v; I/V

Table 6.2 Advantages and disadvantages of different fluid therapy

Route	Advantages	Disadvantages
Oral	• Can be done by owner at home so hospitalisation of patient may not be necessary	• Time consuming • Not all fluids can be administered orally • If there is loss of gastrointestinal function, fluid may not be absorbed from GI tract • Unable to administer large quantities of fluid
Subcutaneous	• Useful in animals with a small bodyweight where other routes are not possible	• Fluid takes at least 30 minutes to be absorbed from injection site • Administration is often painful • Only small amounts can be administered at each injection site • Complications at injection site possible
Intraperitoneal	• A useful site in early shock • Useful in animals with a small bodyweight	• Fluid takes at least 20 minutes to be absorbed from injection site • Complications at injection site possible
Rectal	• Large amounts of non-sterile fluid can be administered	• Cannot be used in cases where the GI tract is unable to absorb fluids • Often poorly tolerated by patient
Intraosseous	• Can be used when peripheral veins are not available • This route is viable in circulatory collapse	• Osteomyelitis is a possible complication • Contraindicated in septic shock, fracture sites and pneumatic bones in birds
Intravenous	• Fluid is administered directly into the circulatory system, where it is needed • Large volumes of fluid can be administered • Short amount of time for fluid to take effect	• Specialised equipment required for administration • Patient must be hospitalised • Patient requires regular monitoring • Risk of overhydration • Possibility of patient interference • Possibility of infection introduced into the vein

Oral administration

If an animal is able to drink voluntarily, the oral route should be used. The owner is often able to encourage the animal to take fluids by mouth at home, avoiding hospitalisation. Commercial isotonic or hypotonic fluids are available: these contain water and electrolytes and can be either drunk voluntarily, syringed into the animal's mouth or administered via a feeding tube. In cases of severe dehydration, however, not enough fluid can be given to correct losses by the oral route. Also, in dehydration there is a loss of gastrointestinal function and fluid is not absorbed efficiently. Finally, not all fluids can be administered orally – another administration route must be used.

Subcutaneous administration (s.c.)

Fluid may be administered subcutaneously. This is not often the route of choice because the fluid takes at least 30 minutes to be absorbed from the injection site. In cases of shock, this time will be even longer. Only small volumes of fluid can be administered s.c. at each injection site as the area becomes painful. A skin slough or infection at the injection site is a possible, but rare, complication.

Subcutaneous fluids are however often useful in animals of very small bodyweight. In these patients, other routes may not be possible or practical. Subcutaneous fluids are also used to maintain fluid levels once rehydration has been achieved, and have been used in the long term to support cats with chronic renal failure.

Intraperitoneal administration (i.p.)

Intraperitoneal fluids are used occasionally in mild dehydration of small patients. The blood vessels in the peritoneum remain dilated until the later stages of shock, so the i.p. route can be used early in the condition. Absorption of fluid from the injection site takes approximately 20 minutes. Complications of this injection site are also possible, e.g. accidental injection into viscera.

Rectal administration

Rectal administration is not possible in cases where the gastrointestinal tract is unable to absorb fluids. Vomiting, diarrhoea and shock will all prevent fluid from being absorbed efficiently from the rectum. Whilst large amounts of non-sterile fluid can be administered rectally, the route is not well tolerated by small animals and is used infrequently.

Intraosseous administration (i.o.)

Intraosseous administration of fluid is useful and is often used when peripheral sites are not available, e.g. due to circulatory collapse. The bone marrow remains unaffected in circulatory collapse because the veins in bone marrow drain into the systemic venous system. Intraosseous

■ Fluid therapy

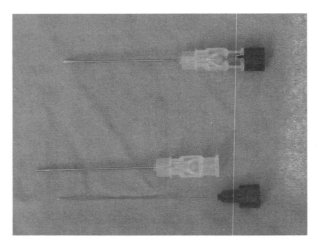

Figure 6.1 Spinal needles (20 G) suitable for intraosseous fluid administration.

fluid administration is sometimes used in neonates and small breeds of dog where catheterisation of a peripheral vein is difficult due to the small size of the vein.

Intraosseous catheterisation is contraindicated in septic shock, in fractured bones and in pneumatic bones of birds. Sites that are used are the tibial crest, the inter-trochanteric fossa of the femur, wing of the ilium, tibial tuberosity and greater tubercule of the humerus. This route can accept large volumes of whole blood, colloids and crystalloid fluids. Intraosseous administration is discontinued once the patient has an intravenous route available, since osteomyelitis is a potential complication of i.o. fluid administration.

An intraosseous catheter or a 20 G spinal needle, as shown in Figures 6.1 & 6.2, is required for i.o. administration.

Steps in intraosseous catheter placement

1. Position the patient with the site to be used easily accessible.
2. Clip the hair using either electric clippers (preferred) or scissors.
3. Prepare the site with surgical scrub.
4. Introduce 1% lignocaine solution (local anaesthetic) into surrounding skin, tissue and periosteum.
5. A small stab incision is made in the skin over the site where the intraosseous catheter is to be introduced, (this prevents blunting of the i.o. catheter).
6. Grasp the bone into which the i.o. catheter is to be inserted.

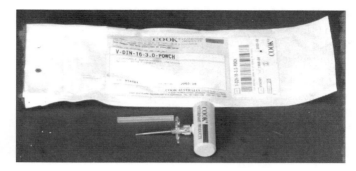

Figure 6.2   Intraosseous needle manufactured by Cook Veterinary Products.

7. The catheter is introduced into the bone using a twisting motion. As soon as the catheter is advanced through the cortex it should slide down into the bone marrow cavity.
8. Advance the needle to the hub.
9. Flush the catheter with heparinised saline.
10. Connect a giving set to the i.o. catheter.
11. Secure the i.o. catheter using zinc oxide tape or by suturing the hub of the catheter to the skin.
12. Place a bandage over the catheter.

Nursing care of the intraosseous catheter is the same as for intravenous catheters.

Intravenous administration (i.v.)

Intravenous administration of fluid has the main advantage that fluid is being administered directly into the circulatory system, where it is needed most. Large volumes of fluid can be administered i.v. over a short period of time. Specialised equipment is necessary to administer fluid i.v. and the patient must be monitored adequately; there is a small risk of overhydrating the patient. However, the advantages of speedy administration directly into the vascular space outweigh the disadvantages. Note that blood and blood products can *only* be administered either intravenously or via the intraosseous route.

Peripheral veins are typically used to administer i.v. fluids – commonly, the cephalic or saphenous veins are used. The cephalic vein is on the cranial aspect of the distal forelimb and the saphenous vein is the lateral aspect of the hock. Less commonly, a central vein – the jugular, on the lateral neck – is used for this i.v. administration. Personal preference determines which vein is used, however the jugular vein has the largest diameter so greater volumes of fluid can be administered in a shorter time via this route.

A wide choice of needles and catheters is available to deliver fluid therapy into the chosen vein:

- Hypodermic needles
- Butterfly needles/scalp vein sets
- Through-the-needle catheters
- Over-the-needle catheters.

Hypodermic needles

Hypodermic needles are *not* recommended for long-term intravenous fluid administration. They are sharp and, if left in the vein, are likely to damage the wall of the blood vessel, causing fluid to leak perivascularly. Hypodermic needles can also easily become dislodged from the vein.

Butterfly needles/scalp vein sets

A butterfly needle (Fig. 6.3) is easy to place in the vein but is more difficult to stabilise than a catheter. As with the hypodermic needle, the butterfly type is sharp and may puncture the wall of the blood vessel.

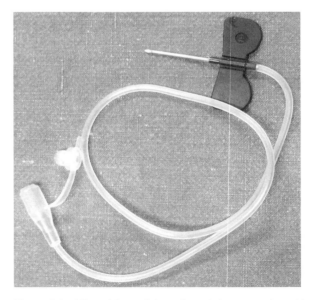

Figure 6.3 Winged 'butterfly' needle and short extension tubing.

Butterfly needles are suitable for the administration of a large bolus of fluid into the vein in one dose, but are best not left in position for any length of time.

Over-the-needle intravenous catheters

Over-the-needle (OTN) catheters are the preferred means for intravenous fluid administration. This type of catheter is easy to stabilise and secure and the catheter remaining in the vein is blunt and unlikely to irritate or puncture the vessel wall. The catheter also has a large lumen through which fluid can easily be administered in large volumes.

The over-the-needle catheter is a length of plastic tubing with a Luer mount at one end. Running inside this catheter is a metal stylet (Fig. 6.4). The stylet is shaped similarly to a needle at one end and this is exposed through the end of the catheter. The stylet stiffens the catheter and the sharp end pierces the skin and wall of the vein at insertion, making introduction easier. Once the catheter is positioned correctly in the vein, the metal stylet is withdrawn to leave only the plastic catheter in the vein. The end of the catheter remaining outside the vein has a Luer mount to which a three-way tap or fluid giving set is attached. An over-the-needle

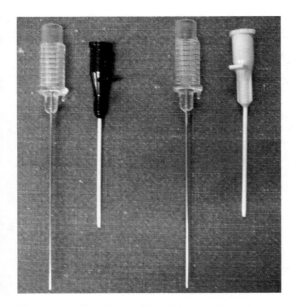

Figure 6.4 Over-the-needle catheters are the preferred means of delivering i.v. fluids. Various sizes and lengths are available. The stiffening metal stylets are shown removed on the left of the two catheters.

Table 6.3 Advantages and disadvantages of hypodermic needles, catheters and butterfly needles

Type	Advantages	Disadvantages
Hypodermic needle	Readily available	Not recommended for long-term i.v. fluid therapy Damage to wall of blood vessel likely Easily dislodged from vein
Butterfly needles/ scalp vein sets	More easily placed than a catheter Useful for administration of large bolus of fluid rather than being left *in situ*	More difficult to stabilise than a catheter Damage to wall of blood vessel likely Easily dislodged from vein
Intravenous catheters	Easily stabilised in the vein Do not cause irritation to the vein Do not puncture the wall of the vein Large lumen allowing high volume of fluid through Damage to wall of blood vessel less likely	More expensive Requires skill in catheter placement Aseptic technique required during placement of catheter Infection possible

catheter can be left in place for up to 48 hours but should then be replaced – this is to prevent thrombophlebitis and infection. This catheter is preferred by many veterinary surgeons over the previously discussed alternatives (Table 6.3). Note that all intravenous catheters must be placed and maintained using an aseptic technique. Prevention of infection being introduced into the circulatory system is vital.

Intravenous catheters are available in different sizes. The diameter of the catheter is expressed as a gauge, for example 23 gauge. The smaller the diameter of the catheter, the *higher* the gauge number. Some manufacturers colour code their catheters according to size, however there is not a universal colour coding system so the individual sizes must be noted rather than the colours. The length of the catheter is expressed in inches or millimetres. The longest, largest diameter catheter possible should be used for two reasons:

1. The longer length makes it more stable when in the vein
2. The wider gauge allows fluid to flow more freely through it, reducing the likelihood of blockage.

However when selecting a long catheter, take care that it isn't so long, or positioned so highly on the leg, that the catheter is kinked near a joint.

Box 6.1	Sizes of intravenous catheter and examples of use
Size of catheter	**Example of breed/species**
24 G	Kitten/puppy and very small dogs, e.g. Chihuahua
22 G	4 kg cat and small dogs, e.g. Jack Russell
20 G	Medium sized dogs, e.g. Spaniel
18 G	25 kg dog, e.g. Labrador
16 G	Giant breed, e.g. Irish Wolfhound

Steps in over-the-needle intravenous catheter placement (Fig. 6.5)

1. Wash hands.
2. Restrain the patient in standing, sternal or lateral recumbency with the vein to be used exposed.
3. Clip hair from vein using either electric clippers (preferred) or scissors. If using scissors always cut at a 45° angle across the vein rather than parallel to it, to reduce the risk of cutting the vein with the scissors.
4. Raise the vein to identify its position.
5. Prepare the site with surgical scrub.
6. Release the vein.
7. Tent the skin overlying the vein and make a small incision over the vein site using the tip of a scalpel blade. This makes insertion of the catheter smoother.
8. Raise the vein again.
9. Introduce the i.v. catheter into the vein. If the catheter is in the vein, blood will be seen in the hub of the catheter – this is known as flash back.
10. Stabilise the stylet and at the same time introduce the catheter into the vein along its length.
11. Connect the three-way tap to the i.v. catheter.
12. Secure the catheter in place using strips of zinc oxide tape cut to size.
13. Flush with 1 mL heparinised saline.
14. Connect the giving set to the three-way tap and turn on the fluid supply.
15. Ensure the fluid is running in and the vein is not 'blown'.
16. Further secure the i.v. catheter in place with strips of zinc oxide tape.
17. Place a bandage over the i.v. catheter.
18. Place the patient in its kennel.

19. Place the fluid bag on a drip stand at least 50 cm higher than the patient to ensure that fluid flows easily.

Having previously calculated the amount of fluid to be given, and at what speed, adjust the drip rate on the giving set to give the required flow (alternatively, programme the infusion pump – Fig. 6.12, p. 67).

Through-the-needle intravenous catheters

Through-the-needle catheters are usually reserved for placement in the jugular vein since they are very long, the length enabling the catheter to be kept in place easily. The catheter has a blunt tip and is unlikely to puncture the blood vessel wall. A through-the-needle catheter is the preferred type for monitoring central venous pressure (see Ch. 2).

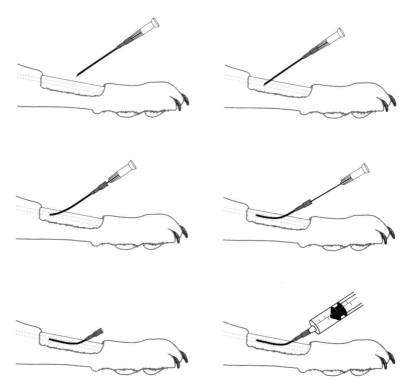

Figure 6.5 Placement of an over-the-needle i.v. catheter. **A, B** The catheter tip (plus stylet) is introduced into the vein. Check for 'flash back' of blood. **C, D** The catheter is advanced into the vein along the stylet. **E** The stylet has been completely withdrawn. **F** The catheter is flushed with heparinised saline and secured using zinc oxide tapes.

The needle has a large lumen and the catheter runs through this, hence the name (Figs 6.6. & 6.7). There are various types of through-the-needle i.v. catheter available and the Seldinger type and placement technique is often used. The Seldinger through-the-needle catheter has a guide wire and dilator to aid insertion of the catheter (Fig. 6.8).

Steps in jugular catheter placement using the Seldinger technique

1. Wash hands.
2. Restrain the patient in either standing, sternal or lateral recumbency with the vein to be used exposed.

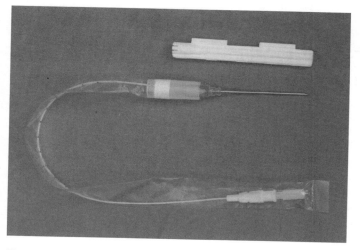

Figure 6.6   A through-the-needle catheter for jugular vein placement.

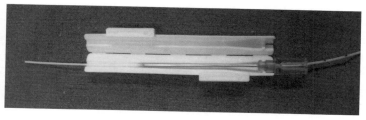

Figure 6.7   The plastic needle guard of a through-the-needle catheter. Once inserted, the needle is withdrawn but cannot be removed from the assembly completely; the needle guard snaps over the needle and protects the patient.

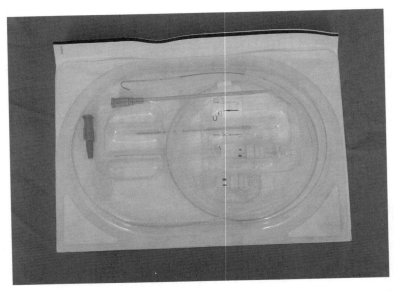

Figure 6.8 A Seldinger set for catheter placement. It incorporates needle, guide wire, dilator and catheter in a sterile single use set.

3. Clip hair from vein using either electric clippers (preferred) or scissors. If using scissors always cut at a 45° angle across the vein rather than parallel to it to reduce the risk of cutting the vein with the scissors.
4. Raise the vein to identify its position.
5. Prepare the site with surgical scrub.
6. Release the vein.
7. Wash hands again and put on sterile surgical gloves.
8. Place a fenestrated drape over the insertion site.
9. Tent the skin and push the needle through the skin, introducing it into the jugular vein.
10. Feed the guide wire through the needle into the vein.
11. Remove the needle, leaving the guide wire in place in the vein.
12. Feed the dilator over the guide wire and into the vein.
13. Remove the dilator.
14. Feed the catheter over the guide wire, without letting go of the guide wire.
15. Remove the guide wire and connect a three-way tap to the catheter.
16. Flush the catheter with 1 mL heparinised saline.
17. Suture catheter in place.
18. Place a bandage over the intravenous catheter.

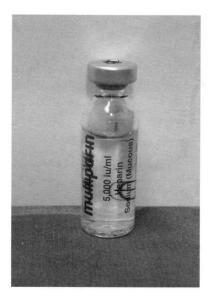

Figure 6.9   Heparin stock vial for making heparinised saline.

General catheter care

The i.v. catheter should be checked at least four times daily. Look for swelling around the insertion site, leakage of fluid from the catheter, dislodging of the catheter and patient interference.

The catheter is bandaged once secured in place in the vein. This helps hold the catheter in position, helps prevent patient interference and keeps the catheter site clean. To do this, place two swabs over the catheter and under the three-way tap to prevent friction and movement. Bandage over this using a light bandage, forming a loop with the giving set and bandaging this to the patient's leg. The loop will take the strain should the animal put a lot of tension on the giving set, thus preventing disconnection from the i.v. catheter. Sometimes a splint is also used to keep the patient's leg in an extended position – this is especially useful in very short-legged breeds such as the Dachshund.

The i.v. catheter should be flushed with heparinised saline after each bag of fluid is given and after an i.v. injection is given. This will maintain a free flow of fluid through the catheter. Heparinised saline is prepared by adding 5 mL of the stock solution of heparin (1000 i.u./mL) to 500 mL of sterile saline (Fig. 6.9).

Box 6.2   General catheter care

Check for swelling around the catheter site

Check for leakage of fluid from the catheter and giving set

Check for dislodgement of the catheter from the vein

Check for a 'blown' vein

Check for patient interference

Check bandage is in place over the catheter

Flush with heparinised saline

Check position of patient's limb

If the fluid stops flowing through the catheter several checks should be made:

- The position of the animal's leg should be checked. If the leg is flexed it may block the flow of fluid.
- The vein must be checked to see if it has 'blown' – this indicates fluid has leaked perivascularly. Signs of a 'blown' vein are swelling over the vein just above the catheter insertion site, patient discomfort and swelling of the limb.
- The level of fluid in the bag should be checked to ensure it has not run out.
- The catheter should be flushed with heparinised saline – this will unblock the catheter.
- The giving set should be checked to ensure it is not kinked and the flow of fluid compromised.
- The catheter position should be checked for patient interference.
- The point at which the catheter joins the giving set should be checked to ensure a secure connection.

Ancillary equipment used in administration of fluid therapy

A range of equipment is used in administering fluid therapy and veterinary nurses should be familiar with these items.

Fluid giving sets

Several types of giving set are in common use:

- Standard fluid giving set
- Blood giving set
- Burette
- Extension set.

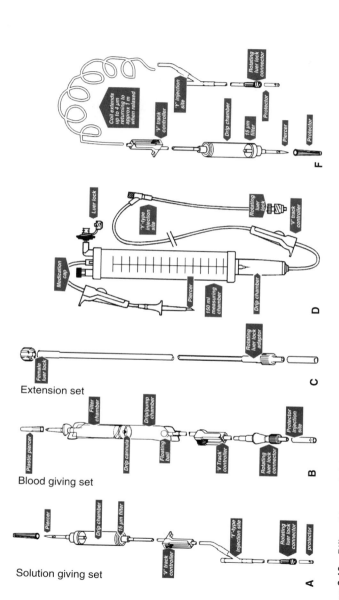

Figure 6.10 Different types of giving set. **A** Standard crystalloid giving set. **B** Blood giving set. **C** Extension sets are useful for active patients in larger kennels. **D** Burettes allow accurate administration of small volumes to low bodyweight patients. **E** The coiled extension tubing in this set allows for movement without entanglement of the extension tubing. (Diagrams reproduced from *The Animalcare Veterinary Infusion and Accessories Range* leaflet, by kind permission of Animalcare Ltd, Dunnington, York.)

All giving sets administer fluid to the patient from the reservoir bag via an intravenous catheter. An alternative name for the giving set is 'fluid administration set'. Giving sets comprise a length of sterile plastic tubing, having a Luer fitting at one end and a spike connection that fits into the fluid bag at the other end. There are two principal types of giving set: one through which crystalloid and colloid solutions are administered, and one through which blood is administered. The blood giving set has a filter incorporated in it since clots must be filtered out before entering the recipient vein. The packaging of each giving set will state its use but the veterinary nurse must be able to recognise the difference between types.

The basic construction of all giving sets is similar, though they may vary in appearance. Some screw into the intravenous catheter, others lock in; some giving sets have an injection port, others do not. A coiled giving set has the advantage of not becoming twisted and kinked – it has more ease of movement with the patient. Some giving sets have a dial flow regulator situated just below the drip chamber which is set to the required mL of fluid to be administered per hour. A new giving set is used for each patient and is discarded after use. Giving sets should also be changed every 24 hours.

A standard giving set will administer either 15 or 20 drops per mL of fluid. This information is printed on the outside of the packaging of the giving set. If this information is not readily available, the manufacturer of the giving set should be contacted and the administration rate checked. It is important the veterinary nurse is aware of the number of drops per mL the giving set administers since this information is needed when calculating flow rates.

Connecting the giving set to the fluid bag

1. Wash hands.
2. Check expiry date on bag of fluid.
3. Examine the fluid bag for particles, leaks and cloudiness. If these are present the bag should be discarded and an alternative selected.
4. Warm the fluid to 37°C by either placing in a bowl of warm water, gently heating in a microwave, using a fluid warming jacket or storing fluids in an incubator.
5. Peel open outer packaging of fluid bag.
6. Hang bag of fluid on a drip stand.
7. Twist off the wings of the giving set port on the bag of fluid.
8. Take giving set from outer packaging, ensuring the two ends of the tubing are not allowed to fall onto the floor or table and thus become contaminated.
9. Turn off the giving set.

10. Insert the spike end into the giving port of the bag of fluid using a gentle half twisting motion.
11. Squeeze the fluid collection chamber two or three times to part fill it with fluid.
12. Turn on the giving set and allow fluid to flow through the full length of the giving set to remove any air from the tubing. Do not allow too much fluid to run through the giving set but all air must be removed from the tubing to prevent air being introduced into the patient's vein, causing an air embolism. There must be no air bubbles in the giving set.
13. Hang the end of the giving set over the drip stand ready for use.

Burettes

A burette is very similar to a standard fluid giving set but has a large graduated collecting chamber along its length. This is extremely useful in smaller patients when a small, accurate amount of fluid is to be given. The fluid flows from the drip bag, along the length of the giving set and is released into a measured collecting chamber (the burette) and then flows along the remaining part of the giving set and into the intravenous catheter (Fig. 6.11).

The burette has measured increments along its length that enable a small amount of fluid, say 50 mL to be given easily. The burette system is useful in cats, small dogs and animals of a low bodyweight where overadministration of fluid could be a problem. The burette is re-filled as necessary from the fluid bag. Burette giving sets administer 60 drops per mL.

Extension sets

An extension set is a length of sterile tubing which can be added to a giving set, should more length be required between the drip bag and the patient. The extension set merely extends the giving set already in use, it has no bearing on the rate of administration. The extension set has Luer connections at each end enabling it to be connected to the standard fluid giving set and the i.v. catheter. An extension set can be useful if the patient is in a wide kennel and may move around, putting too much tension on the shorter giving set.

Infusion pumps

An infusion pump is a piece of equipment that can be used to provide an accurate continuous infusion of fluid, over a set period of time (Fig. 6.12). The pump is connected to the electricity supply and is attached to a drip stand, outside the kennel. A length of giving set is passed through a channel in the door of the infusion pump. The giving set must be of

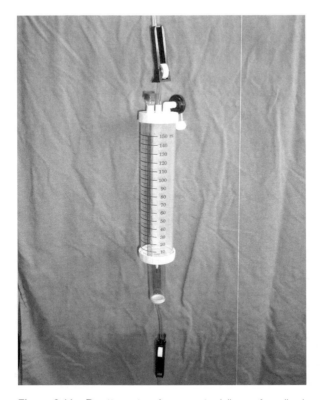

Figure 6.11   Burette system for accurate delivery of small volumes of fluid.

suitable type to be used in the infusion pump: the manufacturer of the pump will recommend the giving set to be used.

The infusion pump is programmed manually to allow a specific number of drops to pass through the tubing in a given amount of time. The veterinary staff will programme in the details, e.g. 100 mL over 60 minutes. An alarm will ring if, for any reason, the fluid is not being administered at the programmed rate. The alarm will be set off if there is a blockage or the drip bag runs out, to illustrate two common problems. The alarm alerts nursing staff immediately a problem arises, enabling prompt attention to be given to the patient.

The infusion pump is an extremely useful piece of equipment since it provides accurate control of fluid administration and immediately informs nursing staff of any deviations. It is not, however, a substitute for regular monitoring of the patient. Infusion pumps are expensive and,

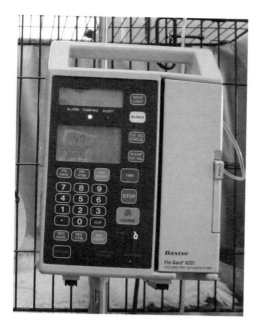

Figure 6.12   An infusion pump fixed to the outside of a hospital kennel.

although useful, are not essential. Indeed, they are beyond the reach of many veterinary practices. When used, however, the fluid rate is undoubtedly controlled more reliably than using a conventional giving set and drip chamber.

Spring-loaded syringes

A more recent development in i.v. fluid therapy equipment is the spring-loaded syringe. These are considerably less expensive and more portable than traditional infusion pumps and are re-usable. The device consists of a spring-loaded cylinder that holds a disposable syringe with intravenous fluid contained in it. The syringe is then connected to a flow-control capillary tube (this tube has been previously calibrated to provide a known set administration rate). The tube connects to the i.v. catheter. A constant rate of infusion is given as the syringe is under pressure from the spring. The flow-control capillary tubes are provided in a variety of dispensing rates and the veterinary staff can select the one suitable for their calculated flow rate.

By administering fluid under pressure, rather than relying on gravity alone as with a conventional giving set, the likelihood of having kinked tubing or a blocked catheter is greatly reduced. The spring-loaded pump fits a 30 mL and 10 mL syringe and is therefore useful for administering a large bolus of an i.v. drug or for fluid administration to exotic species or smaller animals where accurate low volumes are required. The spring-loaded pump can be bandaged onto the patient or laid down beside the animal, depending upon how active the patient is. It can also be attached to the cage by a specifically marketed mounting basket.

The *Flowline*™ supplied by Arnolds (UK) is the spring-loaded syringe many practices use. The system has a refill port attached to the capillary tubing, which enables the syringe to be filled with fluid without disconnecting the equipment (Fig. 6.13).

Pressure bulb syringes

Balloon infusors, marketed by Arnolds (UK), follow a similar principle to spring-loaded syringes. They consist of a sterile latex balloon that is filled with the fluid to be administered. The balloon is then connected to a flow-control tube similar to the type used with the spring-loaded syringe. This provides an accurate amount of fluid given over a set period of time. The balloon is bandaged to the animal or placed on the kennel floor if the patient is recumbent. Fluid is administered under pressure due to the elastic properties of latex. Balloon infusors are single use only and are discarded between patients.

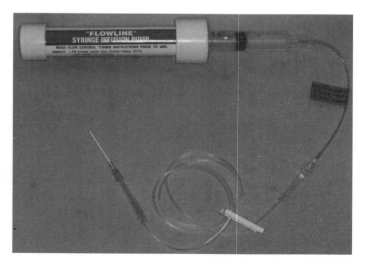

Figure 6.13 Spring-loaded syringe and flow-control tubing (Flowline™ by Arnolds).

Syringe drivers

Syringe drivers are used for administration of i.v. fluids to small animals. The syringe driver delivers a specific volume of fluid over a programmed period of time. A loaded syringe is placed into the syringe driver, and fluid is delivered under pressure at the desired rate (Fig. 6.14). A syringe driver is a very useful means of delivering precise volumes of fluid or drugs to small, critically ill patients.

Ancillary equipment

There are a number of smaller pieces of equipment that, while not essential for i.v. fluid administration, are however useful and should be considered.

A *three-way tap* is useful (Fig. 6.15). This is placed between the i.v. catheter and the giving set. When the patient is initially disconnected from the i.v. line with the catheter left in place, a three-way tap

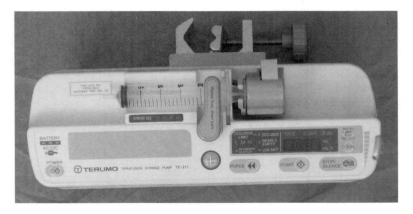

Figure 6.14 A syringe driver is very useful for delivering continuous infusions of drugs or fluids.

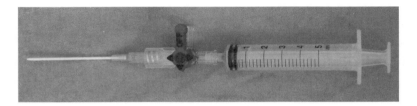

Figure 6.15 5 mL syringe connected to a three-way tap. As assembled, the tap is closed to the side port and open to the attached i.v. catheter.

can also be left *in situ*, providing an instant i.v. route. This makes injection easier than injecting directly into the catheter, with the risk of dislodging it.

A *stopper* or *plug* is useful in bunging the end of the catheter when the giving set is removed (this is used as an alternative to a three-way tap). An i.v. injection can be made through the stopper, enabling the catheter to be flushed regularly.

A *kink resistor* is a commercially available piece of plastic, through which the giving set passes to hold a loop in the giving set without causing kinking.

Heparinised saline is important for regular flushing of the i.v. catheter to prevent blockage. This is prepared by adding 5 mL of the stock solution of heparin (1000 i.u./mL) to 500 mL of sterile saline.

A *T-connector mini extension set* is a small length of extension tubing having a bung port and giving set connection. The T-connector is attached between the i.v. catheter and the standard giving set. It enables drugs to be injected through the bung, which is positioned close to the i.v. catheter. The T-connector also has a white clamp, which must be positioned appropriately to allow fluid to flow through the tubing when fluid is being injected via the bung end. This connector also allows the giving set to be disconnected and yet the i.v. catheter is bunged, which can be useful, e.g. when dogs are taken outside to urinate. It avoids having a long length of giving set and drip bag to handle in an outdoor run.

7

Monitoring the patient on intravenous fluids

Key points

- Overtransfusion is rare in healthy animals but may be seen in those with heart or kidney problems
- Routine monitoring is required for all i.v. patients
- Common causes of interruption in drip flow should be looked out for

---

The patient on intravenous fluid therapy must receive 24 hour nursing care. A fluid monitoring chart should be completed, in addition to the usual hospitalisation records. The fluid monitoring chart can be designed by the veterinary practice to suit their own requirements. All observations and details regarding the animal's fluids should be recorded.

Problems in fluid administration

Overtransfusion

Overloading the animal with fluid during i.v. therapy is a possibility, and will cause oedema (fluid accumulation) in body tissues (Box 7.1). Whilst overtransfusion of i.v. fluids is not common, the patient should be monitored for possible signs. In most cases, should overtransfusion occur,

---

Box 7.1 Signs of overtransfusion

- Increased central venous pressure
- Congestive heart failure
- Collapse
- Dyspnoea
- Depression
- Moist cough
- Tachypnoea
- Pulmonary oedema

---

the kidneys will excrete the excess fluids and restore normal water balance. If there is a pre-existing medical condition, especially heart or kidney disease, then problems with overadministration of fluids are more likely. In general, a maximum infusion rate of 10–15 mL/kg/hour allows rapid correction of fluid imbalances without leading to fluid overload.

The patient should be monitored every 30 minutes as shown in Box 7.2, and the findings recorded on the fluid chart.

Measures taken to avoid overtransfusion

The following procedures can help avoid inadvertent fluid overload:

- Use of a burette or syringe driver in small patients (less than 5 kg)
- Use of an infusion pump for patients not needing a burette or syringe driver
- Careful calculation of the amount and rate of fluid administration
- Accurate history taking
- Repeated patient clinical assessments
- Repeated patient clinical measurements
- Monitoring urine output and comparing this to fluid administration.

As the patient is monitored, an impression of general comfort is gained – this can be an early indicator of fluid overload if the patient becomes quieter or more depressed. Rectal temperature should be recorded. A peripheral pulse rate, if available, should be counted and the strength of

---

Box 7.2 Monitoring the patient on fluids – what to look for

- General well-being
- Temperature
- Pulse rate and strength
- Respiration rate and depth
- Capillary refill time (CRT)
- Colour of mucous membranes
- Urine output of 1–2 mL/kg/hour
- Chest auscultation clear
- Presence of a cough
- Jugular distension
- Packed cell volume (PCV)
- Central venous pressure (CVP)
- Flow rate of fluid
- Patency of i.v. catheter
- Bandage covering i.v. catheter
- Inflammation at catheter site

---

pulse noted. Respiration is likely to increase with fluid overtransfusion. Capillary refill time and mucous membrane colour can easily be checked in most patients; these clinical signs measure cardiac output.

Monitoring the urine output is important in the patient receiving intravenous fluids. Urine output can be measured continuously and accurately if a urinary catheter is in place and a urine collection bag is attached (Fig. 7.1). An indwelling urinary catheter is sited and connected to a urine collection bag. A makeshift urine collection bag can be improvised from an empty fluid bag and giving set. This is connected to the urinary catheter via a three-way tap. Alternatively, the indwelling urinary catheter can have a bung placed in its end and urine drawn off regularly using a syringe and three-way tap.

If a urinary catheter is not in place a rough estimate of the amount of urine passed is made. The animal can be observed urinating and samples

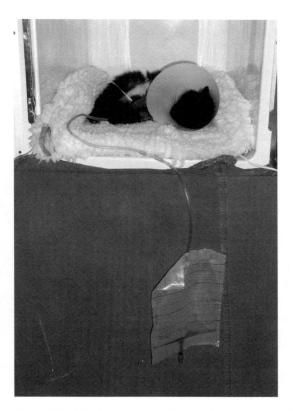

Figure 7.1 Critical care patient with indwelling urinary catheter and collection bag.

collected; bedding wet from urine can be weighed: a 1 g increase in the weight of bedding indicates an approximate loss of 1 mL of urine. These methods are not sufficient in severely compromised patients – accurate measurement of urine is necessary here. Urine output will be restored to normal once the animal becomes re-hydrated. Note that normal urine output is 1–2 mL/kg/hour.

The patient's chest should be auscultated using a stethoscope and any moist chest sounds – râles – should be brought to the attention of the veterinary surgeon immediately. The presence of a moist cough can indicate that the rate of i.v. fluids should be slowed.

Jugular distension is easily felt: this can also be an indication of over-transfusion. Packed cell volume can be measured to assess hydration status: the PCV increases in dehydration so, as the animal receives fluid therapy and its fluid losses are replaced, its PCV should fall. Central venous pressure, if measured (see Ch. 2), can be an indication of the hydration status of the animal.

Monitoring and recording of clinical signs together with these measurements will give a good indication as to the hydration status of the patient. All parameters measured on clinical examination must be recorded and the time of findings also noted. This enables the animal's progress to be followed accurately. All abnormal findings must be reported to the veterinary surgeon immediately.

Interruptions in fluid administration

When monitoring the patient it is important to remember to check the flow rate is sufficient and that there is enough fluid remaining in the bag. The giving set is checked for any kinks or leaks. If kinked, it should be manually untwisted. Coiled giving sets tend to kink less.

If the flow rate has ceased then the source of the problem must be identified. The i.v. catheter may be blocked, in which case it should be

---

Box 7.3   Possible reasons why the drip has stopped

- Fluid bag is empty
- Kinking of giving set
- Blockage of i.v. catheter
- Holes in giving set due to patient interference
- I.v. catheter has become dislodged
- Giving set has become disconnected from the i.v. catheter
- Filter blocked
- Retraction of the limb

flushed with either 5 mL of sterile saline or heparinised saline. The flow rate should then be reset; if the flow is still not running, a new i.v. catheter must be inserted. The catheter may have become dislodged due to either patient interference or the animal moving around excessively in its kennel. Again, a new intravenous catheter should be placed. The patient may have been chewing the giving set so it should be checked for any holes: if any are present, a new giving set can be connected.

Giving sets may become disconnected from the i.v. catheter due to an initial poor connection or because of patient interference. The patient's leg may be wet where fluid has flowed out of the giving set onto the hair and the surrounding bedding may also be damp. The giving set should be reconnected securely and the patient and bedding dried.

The bandage covering the intravenous catheter should be changed at least daily to ensure a clean covering over the i.v. catheter. This also allows the nurse to inspect the catheter site. The patient may chew the bandage or it may easily become soiled – it should be replaced whenever this occurs. An Elizabethan collar can be fitted in patients prone to interfere with their drips.

Information on general catheter care is also provided in Chapter 6.

8

Fluid therapy in large animals

Key points

- Intravenous fluids are used less frequently in large animals
- In cattle, home-made non-sterile fluids may be used – large volumes are required
- Horses require large quantities of sterile, non-pyrogenic fluids
- Hypertonic saline is used relatively frequently in large species
- Electrolyte deficiencies can be important in farm animals

There are significant theoretical and practical differences in fluid therapy techniques between small animals and large animals (cattle, sheep and horses). Since the veterinary nurse may be required to either assist with preparing fluids to administer to these species, or to supervise fluid administration, an understanding of these differences is important.

Requirements for fluid therapy

The clinical situations in which intravenous fluid therapy is required in large animals are relatively few in number. In young adult ruminants (particularly calves), fluids are most commonly administered to correct water and electrolyte losses associated with diarrhoea. The diarrhoea often arises due to viral or bacterial enteritis and a metabolic acidosis due to bicarbonate loss in faeces is a common feature. In adult ruminants, severe enteritis is less common but shock associated with septicaemia or toxaemia is relatively important. A common example is peracute mastitis in lactating cows. Metabolic acidosis secondary to shock is a feature but the primary disturbance is shock due to altered body fluid *distribution* rather than fluid *loss* as such. Adult ruminants also suffer specific disease syndromes that may require treatment with electrolytes (hypocalcaemia, hypomagnesaemia) or glucose (ketosis).

Enteritis is also encountered in foals, although it is less common than in calves and lambs. Foals also occasionally require blood transfusions to manage post-parturient neonatal isoerythrolysis (causing anemia due to red blood cell destruction). Plasma transfusions for failure of passive transfer of antibodies may also be required. In adult equines, fluid therapy is most commonly used in the context of anaesthetic management or treatment of animals with gastrointestinal crises (colic).

Fluid therapy in calves and lambs

This is usually required to manage fluid loss due to enteritis (scours). Typically, these animals have a metabolic acidosis due to bicarbonate loss in diarrhoea. A secondary hypovolaemic shock may be present. When treatment can be initiated prior to the onset of shock, oral rehydration solutions are often effective. A variety of commercial electrolyte mixtures in powder or liquid form intended for dilution in water are available and widely used. These can be offered for voluntary intake (from buckets, bottles or nipple feeders) or by stomach tubing in animals unwilling to drink. It is better to offer such solutions separate from milk feeds, since dilution of milk will prevent normal digestion.

In animals where the disease is more advanced, intravenous fluid therapy is indicated. Because these animals are usually acidotic, a balanced electrolyte solution containing bicarbonate or lactate (Hartmann's solution) is used. The practical aspects of fluid administration in these animals are similar to those for large dogs, although usually a jugular catheter (e.g., 16 gauge over-the-needle) is used rather than one inserted in a peripheral vein. The catheter is sutured in place and covered with a neck bandage. A typical volume of fluid to be given would be 100 mL/kg over 4–6 hours, tailored to the clinical response. As the animal's peripheral perfusion improves, oral fluids are introduced.

Occasionally in very young ruminants, hypoglycaemia is encountered, often as a result of starvation or hypothermia. These animals are treated with parenteral glucose. For practical reasons in lambs this is given by the intraperitoneal route (15 mL of 5% glucose solution for each animal).

Fluid therapy in adult cattle

This is most commonly given as part of the treatment of severe toxaemia, for example associated with toxic (peracute) mastitis. In principle, these cases could be treated in a similar fashion to such diseases in small animals, but often the economical and practical aspects in cattle prevent this. When one considers that a 'shock dose' of fluids for an adult cow (100 mL/kg), would be a total volume of 50 L, the difficulties of applying the same techniques as for small animal patients become apparent. Supplying this volume of isotonic fluid from commercially available infusion bags, which are available in up to 3 or 5 L sizes, is difficult. Two approaches are commonly used to overcome this: preparation

Box 8.1   Preparation of Hartmann's solution

Solution 1

Sodium chloride: 120 g
Potassium chloride: 6 g
Calcium chloride dihydrate: 5.83 g

Use laboratory grade reagents and dissolve in 1 L of sterile water. Can be autoclaved at 15 psi for 15 minutes.

Solution 2

Sodium lactate: 86 mL of 70% syrup
Autoclave at 10 psi for 15 minutes.

When required, mix solutions 1 and 2 and add to 19 L of sterile water.

of home-made isotonic fluid solutions or the use of smaller volumes of hypertonic (concentrated) solutions.

Home-made isotonic solutions

Home-made isotonic fluids are made up according to recipes (see Box 8.1). It is rarely possible to make these either sterile or non-pyrogenic but efforts to reach these ideals should be made. The basic chemicals used (e.g., sodium chloride, salt) should be handled in a clinically clean fashion and water that is as clean as possible should be used (e.g., distilled water if available). Commonly, the practice will have prepared mixtures of the salts in stock and will add these to water when the solutions are required. The solutions can then be administered from a large drum (e.g., a plastic drum from a laboratory supplier) through a large bore giving set into a jugular or ear vein catheter. The drum should ideally be sterilised, but this is rarely practical. An alternative is to use a cold sterilising solution to wash the drum out and then rinse the inside with sterile water before adding the intravenous fluid solution. Dilute bleach has been used for chemical sterilisation.

Various clips and tubes may be required to connect the outlet from the drum to the giving set. A large bore giving set is required to allow appropriately rapid fluid infusion: these are commercially available or else a set intended for blood administration may be used. Dedicated large animal giving sets with a long and coiled tube are ideal and can be anchored to a halter to avoid strain on the catheter. The reservoir is suspended from a pulley above the stall. Alternatively, fluids can be administered under pressure, using a pressurised reservoir such as a device intended for the delivery of chemical sprays. While this allows the rapid infusion of a large volume, it is more difficult to carry out in an aseptic fashion.

Hypertonic solutions

The use of hypertonic solutions is possible in both small and large animals but is more popular in the large species because of the practical and economic difficulties of large volume isotonic fluid administration. The principle of hypertonic saline infusions is to infuse a relatively small volume of concentrated fluid (5–10 mL/kg) that then 'recruits' fluid from the interstitial and intracellular fluid spaces so that it results in a relatively large increase in circulating volume: a plasma expanding effect. The hypertonic fluid may also have other useful effects on blood pressure and circulatory function.

An example of a hypertonic fluid is 9% sodium chloride. This can be made up practically in an aseptic fashion in the practice (e.g., by passing through a bacterial filter) or obtained from a commercial source. Commercially available filters for laboratory use with a pore size of 22 μm or less are suitable but will require the use of a pressure or vacuum system to drive the water across at an acceptable flow rate.

Given the large volumes of isotonic fluids required to restore circulating volumes in adult ruminants, one alternative is to restore plasma volume with a hypertonic solution (7.9%) of normal saline at a dose of 4 mL/kg. It must be realised that the hypertonic saline will only result in a *temporary* improvement in circulating volume and cardiac output. The treatment must be followed up by further fluid therapy to restore total body fluid balance, ideally by the intravenous route but often with oral rehydration solutions in practice.

Fluid therapy in adult horses

Fluid therapy in adult horses is typically used in two circumstances: to treat dehydration and shock or to support blood pressure under anaesthesia. Dehydration may result from enteritis or occasionally from overexertion, especially in hot climates. Shock is usually associated with gastrointestinal crises (colic) or occasionally toxaemia (mastitis, metritis or salmonellosis). Treatment of dehydration and shock is approached in a similar way to that in the small species but, because of the size of the patient, similar practical difficulties are present as in adult cattle. Although it may be attractive to use non-sterile and therefore potentially pyrogenic (fever-causing) fluids in horses, as is sometimes the case with adult cattle, this should be avoided. Horses are more susceptible

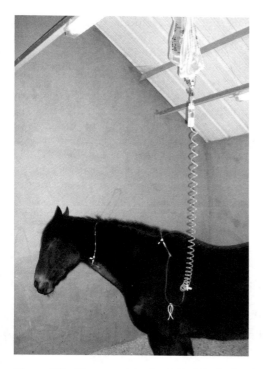

Figure 8.1   Horse receiving i.v. fluids into the jugular vein. A long, coiled extension set allows mobility.

to the potential adverse effects of this technique and, given the often greater monetary or sentimental value of horses, administration of commercially prepared fluids is more appropriate. Three to five litre bags of Hartmann's solution for the treatment of horses are available, together with appropriate large bore coiled giving sets. Some giving sets have two infusion spikes to facilitate simultaneous infusion of multiple bags. Jugular access is routinely used although the lateral thoracic, saphenous, cephalic and median veins are used if the jugulars become thrombotic.

Fluid rates of up to 20 mL/kg/hr (10 L/hr/500 kg horse) of isotonic solutions can be used safely. Hartmann's solution is generally used but in cases of severe documented (i.e., confirmed by blood test) acidosis, sodium bicarbonate solution may be employed. The commercially available stock solution (5 or 8.4%) must be diluted in normal saline before administration.

In hypokalaemic individuals, potassium solution may be used to supplement intravenous fluids at up to 20–40 mmol/L. Calcium supplementation may also be necessary but fluids containing calcium and bicarbonate should not be mixed or given together through the same catheter because they may form precipitates.

For rapid resuscitation, hypertonic saline (7.2%) can be given at 4 mL/kg, administered as rapidly as possible intravenously, but this must be followed up with volume replacement using large amounts of isotonic fluids. Colloids are rarely used in adult horses because of their cost although plasma transfusions are sometimes given to foals. Equine blood will settle into plasma and cells on standing, so centrifugation to separate the major components is not essential. Whole blood transfusions are possible. Ideally, the donor and recipient should be cross-matched. Blood can be collected into commercially available blood bags or into larger containers with anticoagulant added, which should be sterilised.

Electrolyte deficiencies in adult cattle

Calcium, magnesium and phosphorus

Electrolyte deficiencies in adult cattle are relatively common. Around the time of parturition, high yielding milking cows may be affected by hypocalcaemia ('milk fever') or hypophosphataemia. Other adult cattle eating lush grass may become hypomagnesaemic ('staggers') and on occasion different electrolyte abnormalities are present together.

These animals rarely have significant volume deficiencies (dehydration) but require parenteral treatment in the short term to prevent death due to cardiac or other consequences of the electrolyte problems. A range of electrolyte solutions intended for these cases is available, containing the key electrolytes either alone or in combination. Some of these are intended for intravenous use but in others the higher electrolyte levels may be dangerous when administered in this way. Instead, they are given by subcutaneous injection. See Box 8.2.

Electrolyte solutions are often supplied in glass bottles, rather than infusion bags, and require the use of a special giving set ('flutter valve'). This is typically reusable and suitable for autoclaving. A large bore needle is connected to the flutter valve and the fluids given subcutaneously or intravenously. The rate of administration is varied by adjusting the height of the bottle above the animal. Each 400 mL bottle is intended to supply a single dose for a typically affected adult animal.

Hypoglycaemia and ketosis is also encountered in ruminants and may be treated with intravenous 40% glucose (dextrose) solution.

Box 8.2   Typical electrolyte solutions for adult cattle and sheep

Treatment of hypocalcaemia
Calcium borogluconate 40% (equivalent to 3% calcium) for i.v. or s.c. use.

Calcium borogluconate 20% (equivalent to 1.5% calcium) for s.c. use following i.v. treatment.

Treatment of hypomagnesaemia
Magnesium sulphate 25% for s.c. use in divided doses.

Treatment of mixed calcium/magnesium deficiencies
Calcium borogluconate 20% with magnesium hypophosphite 5% for s.c. use in sheep (50 mL/40 kg BW).

Calcium borogluconate 40% with magnesium hypophosphite 5% for i.v. use in cattle.

Treatment of hypophosphataemia
Calcium hypophosphite 4.8% (equivalent to 1.8% phosphorus) for i.v. use.

Multiple choice questions

Choose the most appropriate answer to each question. Answers are on page 89.

1. The daily fluid requirement for an 8 kg dog at twice maintenance is:
   a. 320 mL
   b. 800 mL
   c. 1500 mL
   d. 1750 mL

2. The following is used to measure central venous pressure in the dog:
   a. Over-the needle catheter, 22 G × 1.5″
   b. Scalp vein set
   c. Through-the-needle catheter
   d. Butterfly needle

3. The following should *not* be used in the intraperitoneal route of fluid replacement in a rabbit:
   a. Lactated Ringer's (Hartmann's)
   b. Ringer's
   c. 0.9% sodium chloride
   d. 1.8% sodium chloride

4. If a 24 kg dog appears to be 8% dehydrated, it will require:
   a. 764 mL
   b. 900 mL
   c. 1.43 L
   d. 1.92 L

5. The following statement is true:
   a. Packed cell volume will generally increase in dehydration
   b. Total plasma protein will decrease in dehydration
   c. Creatinine will decrease in dehydration
   d. Bodyweight will increase in dehydration

6. The following is a cause of potassium depletion in a dehydrated animal:
   a. Diabetes insipidus
   b. Urethral obstruction
   c. Vomiting
   d. Addison's disease

7. The following causes an increase in pH of blood:
   a. Removing hydrogen ions from the body
   b. Adding carbon dioxide to the body
   c. Removing bicarbonate ions from the body
   d. Adding hydrogen ions to the body

8. The following results in
   metabolic acidosis:
   a. Chronic vomiting
   b. Cerebral oedema
   c. Chronic diarrhoea
   d. Muscle damage

9. A 40 kg Dobermann is to
   receive intravenous fluids at
   50 mL/kg over a 4 hour
   period. The volume required
   each hour is:
   a. 500 mL
   b. 750 mL
   c. 1500 mL
   d. 2000 mL

10. The circulating blood volume
    of a 4 kg cat is:
    a. 50 mL
    b. 200 mL
    c. 320 mL
    d. 360 mL

11. A 12.5 kg dog has been
    vomiting for 3 days and is
    estimated to be 8% dehy-
    drated. The approximate
    fluid volume you should give
    to rehydrate this dog is:
    a. 500 mL
    b. 1000 mL
    c. 2000 mL
    d. 2240 mL

12. If you wished to maintain a
    36 kg dog on a drip and you
    needed to give 2160 mL
    over 24 hours (assume
    1 mL = 20 drops), you will
    set the drip rate to:
    a. 1 drop per second
    b. 1 drop every 2 seconds
    c. 1 drop every 3 seconds
    d. 2 drops per second

13. A 4 kg cat normally has a
    PCV of 37% but has
    become dehydrated and
    now has a PCV of 44%. For
    rehydration it requires:
    a. 140 mL
    b. 200 mL
    c. 240 mL
    d. 280 mL

14. The daily fluid requirement
    for an 8 kg dog at twice
    maintenance is:
    a. 320 mL
    b. 800 mL
    c. 1500 mL
    d. 1750 mL

15. If a 15 kg dog is found to be
    dehydrated and its present
    PCV is 55%, to replace the
    deficit it requires:
    a. 150 mL
    b. 250 mL
    c. 1500 mL
    d. 3000 mL

16. During i.v. fluid therapy, urine
    output should be maintained
    at:
    a. 1–2 mL/kg/hour
    b. 5–10 mL/kg/hour
    c. 20–30 mL/kg/hour
    d. 56–60 mL/kg/hour

17. The following rises in
    dehydration:
    a. Urine specific gravity
    b. Urine glucose levels
    c. Urine blood levels
    d. Urine ketone levels

18. A cation is:
    a. An ion with a negative
       charge

b. An ion with a positive charge
c. Fluid with an equal pressure to body fluids
d. Fluid with a lower osmotic pressure than body fluids

19. Typically, a burette delivers:
a. 10 drops/mL
b. 15 drops/mL
c. 20 drops/mL
d. 60 drops/mL

20. How many mg/mL are there in a 4% solution?
a. 0.4 mg
b. 4 mg
c. 40 mg
d. 400 mg

21. The following is an example of a crystalloid:
a. Gelofusin
b. Dextran
c. Haemaccel
d. Hartmann's solution (lactated Ringer's)

22. The percentage of a normal adult healthy animal's bodyweight which is water is:
a. 20%
b. 30%
c. 60%
d. 90%

23. The following is an example of an inevitable water loss:
a. Respiratory loss
b. Faecal loss
c. Urinary loss
d. Normal loss

24. Normal maintenance requirements of fluid are:
a. 10–20 mL/kg/24 hours
b. 20–30 mL/kg/24 hours
c. 50–60 mL/kg/24 hours
d. 80–90 mL/kg/24 hours

25. Plasma water represents:
a. >1% of ECF
b. 5% of ECF
c. 15% of ECF
d. 40% of ECF

26. Fluid inside the cells of the body is termed:
a. Intravascular fluid
b. Intracellular fluid
c. Extracellular fluid
d. Plasma water

27. The following is not part of extracellular fluid:
a. Plasma water
b. Interstitial fluid
c. Transcellular fluid
d. Intracellular fluid

28. Synovial fluid is an example of:
a. Extracellular fluid
b. Plasma water
c. Intracellular fluid
d. Interstitial fluid

29. An obese animal will have its bodyweight made up of approximately:
a. 20% fluid
b. 50% fluid
c. 70% fluid
d. 90% fluid

30. The principal electrolyte in intracellular fluid is:
a. Sodium
b. Bicarbonate

c. Chloride
d. Potassium

31. An example cause of primary water loss is:
a. Pyometra
b. Vomiting
c. Starvation
d. Ascites

32. One cause of hypokalaemia is:
a. Vomiting
b. Ruptured bladder
c. Feline lower urinary tract disease (FLUTD)
d. Acute renal failure

33. After tenting, skin should return to its normal position in the healthy animal after:
a. 1 second
b. 2 seconds
c. 5 seconds
d. 6 seconds

34. Normal capillary refill time is:
a. <1 second
b. <2 seconds
c. <5 seconds
d. <6 seconds

35. The clinical signs of dehydration are not detectable until:
a. 5% dehydration
b. 8% dehydration
c. 12% dehydration
d. 15% dehydration

36. 1 kg of water is equivalent to:
a. 250 mL
b. 1000 mL
c. 1500 mL
d. 2000 mL

37. In order to measure central venous pressure, an intravenous catheter is placed into the:
a. Right jugular artery
b. Right jugular vein
c. Left jugular artery
d. Left cephalic vein

38. Central venous pressure in the normal healthy animal measures:
a. 3–7 mmol of water
b. 3–7 L of water
c. 3–7 mm of water
d. 3–7 cm of water

39. A common anticoagulant found in a blood collection bag is:
a. EDTA
b. Heparin
c. CPD
d. Ox F

40. Hartmann's solution is also known as:
a. Ringer's solution
b. Darrow's solution
c. Glucose-saline
d. Lactated Ringer's solution

41. An animal will typically require a blood transfusion if its packed cell volume falls below:
a. 10%
b. 20%
c. 30%
d. 40%

42. The following is used to administer a small

accurate volume of fluid
to a kitten:
a. Blood administration set
b. T-connector
c. Extension set
d. Burette

43. Normal urine output is:
   a. 1–2 mL/kg/hour
   b. 20 mL/kg/hour
   c. 20 mL/kg/24 hours
   d. 50–60 mL/kg/24 hours

44. The most common indication
for fluid therapy in calves is:
   a. Pneumonia
   b. Hypoglycaemia
   c. Scours
   d. Acidosis

45. The usual site of catheter
placement in the horse is:
   a. Saphenous vein
   b. Metatarsal vein
   c. Ear vein
   d. Jugular vein

46. A dose of hypertonic saline
for treatment of shock is:
   a. 1–2 mL/kg
   b. 5–10 mL/kg
   c. 40–50 mL/kg
   d. 90–100 mL/kg

47. A common electrolyte
abnormality in the adult
bovine is:
   a. Hyperphosphataemia
   b. Hypoglycaemia
   c. Hyperkalcaemia
   d. Hypomagnesaemia

48. The following is *not* a
suitable source of water
for home-made intravenous
fluids:
   a. Distilled water
   b. Tap water
   c. Bottled water
   d. Laboratory filtered
   water

49. The ear vein is commonly
used for intravenous fluid
therapy in the:
   a. Dog
   b. Cat
   c. Bovine
   d. Equine

50. 'Staggers' is the colloquial
name for:
   a. Hypocalcaemia
   b. Hypercalcaemia
   c. Hypomagnesaemia
   d. Hypermagnesaemia

Answers to multiple choice questions

1. b, 2. c, 3. d, 4. d, 5. a, 6. c, 7. a, 8. c, 9. a, 10. b
11. b, 12. b, 13. d, 14. b, 15. c, 16. a, 17. a, 18. b, 19. d, 20. c
21. d, 22. c, 23. a, 24. c, 25. b, 26. b, 27. d, 28. a, 29. b, 30. d
31. c, 32. a, 33. b, 34. b, 35. a, 36. b, 37. b, 38. d, 39. c, 40. d
41. b, 42. d, 43. a, 44. c, 45. d, 46. b, 47. d, 48. c, 49. c, 50. c.

Further reading

Adams W, Niles J 1999 Management of the critical care unit. In: Hotston-Moore A, Simpson G (eds) Manual of advanced veterinary nursing. BSAVA, Gloucester, p 85–112

Anon 2002 Veterinary nursing revision guides – fluid therapy. BVNA, Harlow

Dibartola S P 1992 Fluid therapy in small animal practice. W B Saunders, Philadelphia

King L, Hammond R (eds) 1999 Manual of canine and feline emergency and critical care. BSAVA, Cheltenham

Michell A R et al 1989 Veterinary fluid therapy. Blackwell Science, Oxford

Moore M, Palmer N 2001 Calculations for veterinary nurses. Blackwell Science, Oxford

Orpet H, Welsh P 2002 Handbook of veterinary nursing. Blackwell Science, Oxford

Welsh E 1999 Fluid therapy and shock. In: Lane DR, Cooper B (eds) Veterinary nursing. Butterworth Heinemann, Oxford, p 568–585

Appendix 1

Equivalent values; urine and blood parameters

Equivalent values of common measuring units

Volume

Standard units: litres (L) and millilitres (mL)

1 L = 1000 mL
0.5 L = 500 mL
0.25 L = 250 mL

Weight

Standard units: kilograms (kg), grams (g), and milligrams (mg) and micrograms (μg)

1 kg = 1000 g
0.5 kg = 500 g
1 g = 1000 mg
1 mg = 1000 μg

Weight/volume equivalency

1 mL of water weighs 1 g at 15°C

1000 mL weighs 1000 g
1 L weighs 1 kg

Weight conversions

To convert weight in lbs to weight in kg:

Bodyweight in lbs × 0.45 = bodyweight in kg
e.g. Dog weighs 10 lb.
   10 lb × 0.45 = 4.5 kg

To convert weight in kg to weight in lbs

Bodyweight in kg × 2.2 = bodyweight in lbs
e.g. Dog weighs 20 kg
20 kg × 2.2 = 44 lbs

Temperature conversions

To convert °F to °C

$$°C = (°F - 32) × 0.5555$$

To convert °C to °F

$$°F = (°C × 1.8) + 32$$

Equivalents for clinical temperatures

°C	°F
36.0	96.8
36.5	97.7
37.0	98.6
37.5	99.5
38.0	100.4
38.5	101.3
39.0	102.2
39.5	103.1
40.0	104.0
40.5	104.9
41.0	105.8
41.5	106.7
42.0	107.6

Normal parameters

The following tables give normal values for clinical and laboratory parameters, together with common reasons for higher or lower than normal results.

Urinalysis

Test	Canine normal	Feline normal	Higher result	Lower result
Urine specific gravity (SG)	1.015–1.040	1.015–1.050	Dehydration	Diabetes insipidus; i.v. fluid therapy
pH	5.5–7.0	5.5–7.0	Urinary tract infection; animal eaten recently	Established metabolic alkalosis due to severe vomiting
Protein	Negative/ trace	Negative/ trace	Urinary tract infection; renal disease; pyometra; lymphosarcoma; congestive heart failure	—
Glucose	Negative	Negative	Diabetes mellitus; stress; severe bladder trauma	—
Blood	Negative	Negative	Urinary tract infection; renal trauma; urinary calculi; prostatic disease	—
Bilirubin	Trace	Negative	Bile duct obstruction; liver damage	—
Ketones	Negative	Negative	Liver damage; diabetes mellitus	—

Blood biochemistry

Test	Canine normal	Feline normal	Higher result	Lower result
Total protein	58–73 g/L	69–79 g/L	Dehydration; infection	Protein loss; liver failure
Albumin	26–35 g/L	28–35 g/L	Dehydration	Protein loss; liver failure
Globulin	18–37 g/L	23–50 g/L	Dehydration; infection	Infection
Creatinine	30–90 μmol/L	26–118 μmol/L	Dehydration; renal disease	Muscle wastage
Urea	1.7–7.4 mmol/L	2.8–9.8 mmol/L	Dehydration; renal disease	Liver failure
Glucose	3–5 mmol/L	3.3–5.0 mmol/L	Diabetes mellitus	Sample storage problems; insulin overdose; liver failure
Calcium	2.3–3.0 mmol/L	2.1–2.9 mmol/L	Lymphosarcoma; renal disease; Addison's disease	Eclampsia; hypoparathyroidism; polyuria/polydipsia; vomiting; lethargy
Sodium	139–154 mmol/L	145–156 mmol/L	Dehydration	Overhydration
Potassium	3.6–5.6 mmol/L	4–5 mmol/L	Acute renal disease; urethral obstruction	Anorexia; renal disease; collapse

Haematology

Test	Canine normal	Feline normal	Higher result	Lower result
Packed cell volume (PCV)	39–55% NB (up to 65% in sighthounds)	24–45%	Dehydration	Anemia
Haemoglobin	12–18 g/dL	8–14 g/dL	Dehydration	Anemia
White blood cell count (WBCC)	6–15 × 10⁹/L	7–20 × 10⁹/L	Inflammation; infection	Sepsis
Red blood cell count (RBCC)	5.0–8.5 × 10¹²/L	5.5–10 × 10¹²/L	Dehydration	Anemia

Body temperature

Canine normal	Feline normal	Higher result	Lower result
38.3–38.7°C 100.9–101.7°F	38.0–38.5°C 100.4–101.6°F	Excitement; pain; infection; heat stroke	Shock; circulatory collapse; inflammation; hypothermia

Pulse rates

Canine normal	Feline normal	Higher result	Lower result
60–180 beats per minute	110–180 beats per minute	Fever; excitement; pain; fear	Anaesthesia; sleep; unconsciousness

Respiratory rates

Canine normal	Feline normal	Higher result	Lower result
10–30 breaths per minute	20–30 breaths per minute	Heat; exercise; pain	Sleep

Appendix 2

Glossary of fluid therapy and clinical terms

Term	Meaning
Acidosis	Condition in which the pH of body tissues falls below 7.35
Agglutination	Clumping together of cells or particles
Alkalosis	Condition in which the pH of body tissues rises above 7.45
Anion	Negatively charged ion
Anorexia	Loss of appetite
Ascites	Accumulation of fluid in the abdomen
Aseptic technique	Method to ensure absence of bacteria, fungi, viruses or other pathogenic microorganisms
Atom	Particle that cannot be divided further
Auscultation	Listening to sounds in the body that are transmitted to the surface
Bicarbonate	Electrolyte imbalance with hydrogen ions which determines the acidity of body fluids
Blood grouping	Testing an individual to see whether the blood is compatible with another individual's blood
Buffer	Solution or substance that resists change in pH
Capillary refill time (CRT)	Time taken for mucous membranes to return to their normal pink colour after occlusion
Cation	Positively charged ion
Central venous pressure (CVP)	Pressure within the right atrium of the heart

Clinical examination	Examination of an animal by looking at the patient and measuring parameters such as temperature, pulse, respiration, heart sounds, colour of mucous membranes
Colloid	Substance that, although dissolved, can not pass through a membrane
Cross-match	Test performed on blood to determine the presence of antigens that will cause a reaction between donor and recipient blood
Crystalloid	Fluid consisting mainly of water and some electrolytes; used in fluid therapy
Deficit	Deficiency
Dehydration	Excessive loss of water from the body
Diarrhoea	Copious emptying of the bowel, often producing watery faeces
Drip factor (giving set rate)	Number of drops per mL of fluid delivered by a fluid giving set
Dyspnoea	Difficulty in breathing
EDTA (ethylenediamine tetra-acetic acid)	Anticoagulant used in blood sampling
Effusion	Abnormal outpouring of fluid into tissues or cavities of the body
Electrolyte	Liquid that conducts electricity due to the presence of either positive or negative ions
Extracellular	Outside the cells
Giving set rate (drip factor)	Number drops per mL of fluid delivered by a fluid giving set
Haemoglobinuria	Presence of haemoglobin in the urine
Haemolysis	Destruction or breakdown of red blood cells
Haemorrhage	Escape of blood from a ruptured blood vessel, either internally or externally
Heparin	Anticoagulant used in blood sampling and also used to prevent blood clotting in the body

Hypersalivation	Excessive salivation
Hypertonic	Solution having a greater osmotic pressure than plasma
Hypoglycaemia	Low blood level of glucose
Hypokalaemia	Low blood level of potassium
Hypotonic	Solution having a lower osmotic pressure than plasma
Hypovolaemia	Decrease in the volume of circulating blood/reduced amount of fluid in the vascular compartment
Ileus	Paralysis of intestines
Inevitable (insensible) water loss	Fluids lost during metabolism that cannot be regulated by the body, e.g. panting, sweating
Interstitial	Surrounding the cells
Intracellular	Inside a cell
Intraperitoneal (i.p.)	Into the peritoneal cavity
Intravascular (i.v.)	Into a blood vessel (also means intravenous)
Ion	Electronically charged particle
Isotonic	Solutions having the same osmotic pressure
Jaundice	Staining of tissues due to the accumulation of bilirubin
Lactate	Chemical that can be metabolised by the liver to produce bicarbonate ions; lactate is also a product of anaerobic metabolism in shock
Lateral recumbency	Lying on one side
Luer	Universal size system used for equipment such as the ends of giving sets, catheters, stoppers, syringes, etc., allowing the end of one piece of equipment to connect into another
Maintenance requirements	Minimum amount of fluid an animal requires to maintain life; the amount of

	fluid an animal needs to replace those losses that will always occur, e.g. via respiration
Manometer	Gauge used to measure fluid pressure
Metabolism	Chemical reactions within the body
Oedema	Accumulation of excess fluid in a tissue or body cavity
Oliguria	Production of an abnormally small amount of urine
Osteomyelitis	Infection of the medullary cavity of bone
Overtransfusion	Excess of fluid administered to a patient
Packed cell volume (PCV)	Proportion of blood that is red blood cells
Perfusion	Passage of fluid through a tissue
Peripheral	Outer parts
pH	Measure of the concentration of hydrogen ions in a solution and therefore a measurement of its acidity or alkalinity
Plasma	Fluid component of blood in which the blood cells and platelets are suspended
Pulmonary	Relating to the lungs
Pulmonary oedema	Abnormal accumulation of fluid in the lungs
Pyometra	Accumulation of pus in the uterus
Pyrexia	Body temperature above the normal range
Râles	Moist chest sounds
Rectal	Relating to the rectum
Semipermeable membrane	Cell membrane that allows the passage of some molecules but not others, depending on their size, shape and molecular charge
Skin turgor	Elasticity of skin; whether the skin falls back into its normal position after it has been tented
Solution	Chemical (salt) dissolved in a fluid (water)
Specific gravity	Concentration of a solution

Sternal recumbency	Lying on the sternum (breastbone)
Stylet	Stiffener that is passed through the lumen of a tube, e.g. a catheter
Subcutaneous (s.c.)	Under the skin
Tachypnoea	Increase in respiratory rate
Thrombophlebitis	Inflammation of a vein
Urticaria	Reddened area of oedema on the skin
Vomiting	Violent expulsion of stomach contents via the mouth

Index

Note: Page numbers set in *italics* refer to definitions in the Glossary.